MADNESS:
A BIOGRAPHY

PAUL FALLON

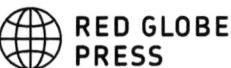

macmillan international HIGHER EDUCATION   RED GLOBE PRESS

First published 2019 by
RED GLOBE PRESS

Red Globe Press in the UK is an imprint of Springer Nature Limited, registered in England, company number 785998, of 4 Crinan Street, London, N1 9XW.

Red Globe Press® is a registered trademark in the United States, the United Kingdom, Europe and other countries.

ISBN 978-1-137-60304-3 paperback

This book is printed on paper suitable for recycling and made from fully managed and sustained forest sources. Logging, pulping and manufacturing processes are expected to conform to the environmental regulations of the country of origin.

A catalogue record for this book is available from the British Library.

A catalog record for this book is available from the Library of Congress.

CONTENTS

List of Figures   vi
Acknowledgements   vii

Introduction   1
1 Anxiety Disorders   5
2 Depression   46
3 Dementia   62
4 Eating Disorders   71
5 Psychosis   94
6 Bipolar Disorder   123
7 Dual Diagnosis   142
Conclusion   150

References   151
Index   164

LIST OF FIGURES

1.1 A woman expressing thanks to the Madonna del Parto for
cure of insanity in the form of expelled devils. Oil painting.
Sansovino, Iacopo, 1486–1570. Madonna del parto.   13

2.1 Robert Burton: *The anatomy of melancholy*; London: Peter Parker,
1676. Frontispiece engraved by C. le Blon.   49

2.2 Portrait of Oliver Cromwell, with facsimile signature by
W. Holl.   51

4.1 Two woodcuts showing Miss C. before and after treatment in
Anorexia Nervosa by William Withey Gull, M.D. published in
Transactions of the Clinical Society of London.   75

5.1 Socrates. Line engraving by P. Pontius, 1638, after
Sir P. P. Rubens.   103

5.2 The hospital of Bethlem [Bedlam] at Moorfields: The entrance
facade. Engraving by A. Soly.   107

5.3 William Norris, shackled on his bed at Bedlam.   111

ACKNOWLEDGEMENTS

When I first explained to my wife Debbie the idea I had for a book on mental health she was very supportive; I then received further encouragement when I discussed it with my friend Jon during our trip to Barcelona to do the marathon. However, it was only after discussing it with Peter Hooper from Red Globe Press that it became a possibility. Peter has been unstinting in his encouragement and support throughout the process and I thank him for that. I'd also like to thank Stanly and his team at Integra for the editing of the manuscript. Also Jon's wife Elaine who as an established author gave me invaluable advice at various stages. This book couldn't have been written if I hadn't worked with so many wonderful staff and patients throughout my nursing career many of whom taught me a great deal about mental health and mental ill health, as well as their causes and effects. For their total and unwavering support I thank Debbie, Natasha and Dan.

Paul Fallon, April 2019.

Introduction

In its updated fact sheet on mental disorders in 2018, the World Health Organization (WHO) estimated that globally 300 million people are affected by depression, 60 million people by bipolar affective disorder, 23 million people by schizophrenia and other psychoses and 50 million people by dementia (WHO, 2018a). In 2018, the WHO also published on its website key facts on suicide and stated that it estimated that 800,000 people die by suicide every year, which is one person every 40 seconds. Furthermore, it stated that suicide was the second leading cause of death among 15–29-year-olds globally in 2016 (WHO, 2018b). While it is not suggested that all of the people who committed suicide had a mental illness, the WHO noted the well-established link between suicide and mental disorders in high-income countries. It also pointed out that suicide isn't just an issue for high-income countries but is a global phenomenon and that over 79 per cent of suicides in 2016 occurred in low- and middle-income countries.

Mental health issues and their consequences are global phenomena affecting people in all regions of the world and in countries of all incomes. Despite this, the WHO also noted that in low- and middle-income countries, between 76 and 85 per cent of people with mental disorders receive no treatment for their disorder and that in high-income countries, between 35 and 50 per cent of people with mental disorders are in the same situation (WHO, 2018a). In fact, the independent Mental Health Taskforce (MHT) (2016) reported to National Health Service England that one in four people in the UK experience mental health problems each year and that up to 75 per cent receive no help, however nearly 2 million adults were in contact with specialist mental health and learning disability services at some point in 2014/15. They estimated the economic and social costs of poor mental health to the UK economy to be £105 billion per annum

(MHT, 2016). Many people with mental health issues are not seen by specialist services but are seen in primary care by their general practitioner (GP), for example, over 57 million antidepressant items were dispensed in the community in 2014, an increase of 7.2 per cent on the previous year (Health and Social Care Information Centre, 2015).

Mental health problems are as old as humanity itself, yet despite this they are still underfunded and under-resourced in health services around the world, being the poor relation in health economies everywhere. They are also still widely misunderstood and in some places treated with fear and superstition – people with these problems are often subject to stigma and, in some places, to outright mistreatment. This book aims to give an introductory explanation of some of the most common and some of the most severe mental health problems including those mentioned above. Each chapter will describe a particular condition or set of conditions (as is the case with anxiety disorders for example) and will then present case studies of historical figures that are generally accepted to have had the condition. The book will try to highlight, via case studies, the different ways that the conditions have been understood at different historical periods and how people with them have been treated both in the sense of by society generally and, specifically, by whatever medical system existed at that particular historic period. When describing a particular condition I will describe the main signs and symptoms to give an overview of the condition. The intention is not to describe every symptom and condition that must be met for a clinical diagnosis of a particular condition to be made. There are two diagnostic manuals, the *American Diagnostic and Statistical Manual* (current version *DSM-V*) and the *European International Classification of Diseases* (current version *ICD-10*), that already seek to fulfil this role. The aim here is to give the reader an understanding of what people with a particular condition are most likely to experience and consequently how they present to others.

The book will then discuss, via contemporary cases, present-day treatments and current debates on the nature of mental health and ill health, including recent developments such as the survivor movement, non-medical approaches to living with mental health difficulties and the growth of the recovery philosophy in mental health services in many areas of the world. It will then highlight how frank discussions of their experiences with mental health difficulties by well-known people is not new but is currently an increasing trend that has begun to have a positive impact on existing efforts by service users, mental health workers and some governments to confront the ignorance, stereotypes and especially the stigma that is all too often attached to mental health issues.

The mental health conditions that will be discussed are: anxiety disorders which will include social anxiety disorder, obsessive compulsive disorder (OCD), panic disorder and trauma induced disorders (from shell shock to post-traumatic stress disorder); depression; dementia; eating disorders; psychosis/schizophrenia; bipolar disorder; and dual diagnosis (individuals with more than one mental health condition or mental health conditions made worse by excessive use of illicit drugs or alcohol). These have been chosen as they comprise the majority of conditions that would be seen in clinical practice today. Each chapter will include a discussion on how these disorders are conceptualised today in diagnostic terms. Controversies that still exist over the validity of some of the diagnostic labels, such as 'schizophrenia', will be discussed in the relevant chapters.

The biographical sketches of individuals throughout history are used to provide information on how the individuals discussed experienced their own particular mental health difficulties within the wider social context of the time in which they were living. This approach makes it possible to compare how societies have changed over time in their attitudes to mental illnesses, how concepts of mental health and ill health have changed and how treatment approaches have developed throughout the ages. The use of a number of brief historical biographies of people from a wide range of backgrounds rather than an in-depth look at a much smaller number of cases has been chosen on purpose to highlight how common mental health difficulties are and also that no one, no matter what status or wealth, is immune to them.

There are, of course, problems with retrospectively diagnosing historical figures with conditions that exist today but that would not have been recognisable to earlier societies, or where similar conditions did exist how they were perceived and what they entailed have changed. For example, people in the Middle Ages did not think of people that were excessively sad or melancholic as 'depressed' as we understand the concept at the moment, and the same is true for people living two centuries ago. What is true, though, is that there are some key features of melancholia that would be recognisable to people who are experiencing a depressive episode today. I have tried to describe how conditions have changed throughout history and have avoided welding on modern concepts to people from earlier times. The use of historical figures who experienced certain symptoms highlights the changing ways in which people have thought about particular mental health conditions.

It has been argued persuasively (Leudar, 2001; Fraguas & Breathnach, 2009) that there are problems labelling people in history who experienced hearing voices as schizophrenic. As a concept, schizophrenia itself has been subject to many different definitions throughout the twentieth century (Fraguas & Breathnach, 2009), showing just how contested a concept it is and how difficult it would be to try to identify people from history as having it, as we currently understand it. However, if we look for descriptions of those deemed mad that encompass symptoms such as hallucinations or delusions then, as Fraguas & Breathnach (2009) have pointed out, many studies have found evidence of schizophrenia-*like* descriptions throughout history and across diverse cultures. All diseases, even physical ones with clearer symptoms and causes than mental health conditions, are historically constructed and as such their descriptions have changed throughout history (Wilson, 2000). One of the dangers of retrospective diagnosis (Wilson, 2000) is that it suppresses the content of past descriptions of conditions; I have attempted to avoid this by explicitly describing the changing nature of the conditions discussed in this book. Sometimes the symptoms that comprise a condition change over time, sometimes whole conditions, whether physical or mental, disappear totally from medical textbooks. Therefore, I am not arguing that the conditions described in this book as they now exist are timeless categories. What I am trying to describe are recognisable human emotions, thoughts, experiences and behaviours that have attracted different descriptions throughout history and are now understood in their current constructions as the conditions discussed in this book.

1

Anxiety Disorders

Experiencing anxiety is a normal part of life and it is something that almost all of us will experience at some point in our lives. Anxiety has a positive function that can be very useful for humans as it readies the body to react to a perceived threat. This is commonly known as the 'fight or flight mechanism' and describes the situation where the autonomic nervous system of humans or other animals is activated in response to a threatening situation. The autonomic nervous system is so called because it acts automatically and it regulates bodily functions including heart rate, respiratory rate, pupillary response and urination. The increase in heart rate increases blood flow to muscles and increases blood pressure to boost the strength and speed of the body, readying it for action.

However, people who have been diagnosed with anxiety disorders frequently have intense, excessive and persistent worry and fear about everyday situations (Cromby et al., 2013). The emotional reaction seems to others to be out of proportion to the actual situation. As well as a cognitive component, i.e. the individual's thoughts, there are also physiological symptoms such as heart palpitations, hot flushes, sweating, hyperventilation, muscle tension and a churning stomach. Anxiety disorders are among the most common of the psychological disorders and research has consistently shown that having a specific phobia (having a fear of a specific situation or thing, for example a fear of spiders, which is termed *arachnophobia*) is the most common type of anxiety disorder that people are likely to experience (Linden, 2012). It has been shown that Obsessive Compulsive Disorder (OCD) is the least common anxiety disorder (Kessler et al., 2010). Most people develop a phobia or OCD in adolescence or early adulthood whereas other anxiety disorders such as panic disorder, agoraphobia and generalised anxiety disorder (GAD) tend to have later and more dispersed ages of onset (ibid.). Post-traumatic stress disorder (PTSD) is an anxiety disorder that occurs in response to a highly traumatic event and, as such events can occur at any time in our lives, PTSD has no link to age.

A significant body of research suggests that if left untreated anxiety disorders are very likely to become chronic in nature and therefore harder to treat (Altamura et al., 2013). It has been argued (Barlow, 2004) that what distinguishes anxiety disorders from major depressive episodes is that depression tends to remit temporarily whether treated or not, whereas anxiety disorders tend to be chronic and remain in a less severe form even when treated successfully. In general, anxiety disorders affect women more than men and this has been found in studies of both developed and a number of developing countries, though the causes of this remain unclear (Craske & Stein, 2016). The World Health Organization (WHO, 2001) has argued that there are several factors that may influence these higher rates in females, noting the close temporal relationship between higher rates of anxiety in women and reproductive age, and that this is also a time in life that is often associated with significant hormonal changes. WHO also noted social, non-biological reasons such as the much higher rate of domestic and sexual violence that women are subjected to; experiences that are also found cross-culturally in societies all around the world.

Anxiety disorders are also influenced by the specific cultural context within which people live – it has been found that different cultures worry about different things and in different ways. Western societies commonly worry about work-related matters whereas in Nigeria, for example, anxiety is often associated with procreation, sterility and impotence; and Inuit communities sometimes experience a panic state while seal-hunting which they term 'kayak angst' (Cromby et al., 2013). There are also some differences in how different cultures experience specific anxiety disorders, for example, in Western societies women are more likely to be diagnosed with agoraphobia (a fear of going outdoors) whereas, in Japan, the similar disorder of *taijin kyofusho* (TKS) is diagnosed equally among men and women (ibid.). In Western societies people often become agoraphobic due to fears around having a panic attack and embarrassing themselves in public whereas, in Japan, people with TKS worry about harming other people, often by emitting noxious odours (ibid.).

It should, however, be noted that some disorders that were once thought to be specific only to certain cultures have turned out to be more common than first thought. An example of this is *dhat syndrome* which was thought to be prevalent mainly in India and is an anxiety disorder in which the sufferer believes they have a loss of semen usually through nocturnal emission, in urine or through masturbation. However, similar anxieties around semen loss have been found to be documented in eighteenth and nineteenth century European, American and Australian literature (Asmal & Stein, 2009) meaning that this particular fear is less 'culture bound' and more widespread than was originally thought.

Generalised anxiety

For many people anxiety can be provoked by many situations and no sooner has one situation been resolved than people then find something else to worry about. This chronic worrying is termed generalised anxiety disorder (GAD) and for someone to be classed as having GAD they must have experienced anxiety and worry about a number of events or activities for more days than not for at least six months (WHO, 2018c). This is accompanied by at least three out of six symptoms which are: restlessness; being easily fatigued; difficulty concentrating or mind going blank; irritability; muscle tension; and sleep disturbance. The anxiety, worry or physical symptoms must also lead to significant distress or impairment in important functional areas (ibid.). For most people the onset of GAD is gradual and most people that get diagnosed with GAD describe having been worried or anxious all their lives (Wells & Butler, 1999). Unsurprisingly, this lifelong tendency to worry about many things in life means that many people with GAD also experience other mental health difficulties, such as social anxiety or depression. People with GAD often feel overwhelmed by trying to cope with all the issues that they are worrying about – at one and the same time they believe worrying about things is a good thing to do because thinking of potential negative consequences prepares them to prevent them yet, they also appraise their tendency to worry in a negative way and hence worry about the fact that they worry so often (ibid.). This makes GAD one of the more complex anxiety disorders and therefore quite difficult to treat.

Panic disorder

Often, anxiety involves repeated episodes of sudden feelings of intense anxiety and fear or terror that reach a peak within minutes accompanied by at least four of the following symptoms: breathlessness; palpitations; dizziness; trembling; nausea; a feeling of chocking; de-realisation; chest pain; and paraesthesia (tingling, numbness or 'pins and needles') (WHO, 2018c). These episodes are known as *panic attacks* and occasional panic attacks are common to all anxiety disorders, however, for an individual to be diagnosed as having panic *disorder* these attacks have to be recurrent and followed by one month or more of persistent worry about future attacks. Often the panic attacks occur in the absence of a trigger and the fact that they can occur unexpectedly makes this an unsettling condition for the person that experiences them. It is the unexpected 'out of the blue' nature of these panic attacks that distinguishes panic disorder from other anxiety disorders that are often accompanied by panic attacks. Panic disorder derives its name from the Greek word *panikon*, meaning "pertaining to Pan," the Greek god who was known for spreading terror.

Phobias

As previously mentioned, specific phobia is the most common type of anxiety disorder (Craske & Stein, 2016) and what makes them a disorder is that the anxiety they provoke is disproportionate to the actual situation or object. It is the exaggerated, or unrealistic, sense of danger that distinguishes a phobia from fear of a situation or object. To avoid this perceived danger, people often organise their lives so that they do not come into contact with the thing that provokes their anxiety. This may have little impact on a person's life if, for example, they are fearful of uncommon objects such as sharks but if one has a complex phobia such as agoraphobia, where the individual may be fearful of open spaces, crowded places or situations it is impossible to escape from easily, such as on public transport, this can have a severe impact on their life. Some people point to the link between agoraphobia and panic disorder, seeing agoraphobia as a strategy to cope with panic attacks by avoiding those situations that the individual thinks will provoke panic attacks (White & Barlow, 2004).

The other main complex phobia is *social anxiety disorder*. This is a marked and persistent fear of social or performance situations due to the individual's belief that they will act in a way that will be embarrassing or humiliating. As with agoraphobia, people try to protect themselves from exposure to the fear by avoiding situations they find fearful. The most common situations are those associated with performance such as public speaking or social situations that involve interacting with others (Clark, 1999). To be diagnosed with social anxiety disorder the symptoms must persist for several months and there must be significant distress and impairment to the person's educational, occupational, social or other important areas of functioning (WHO, 2018c).

The first written references to phobic problems are found in the works of the ancient Greek physician, Hippocrates, who was from the island of Kos and lived between 460 and 370 BCE. These writings were probably the work of a number of authors so it would be more accurate to regard Hippocrates as a collective pseudonym (Pietikainen, 2015) rather than the works of just one man. Hippocrates wrote about a man called Nicanor who, when he went out became terrified of flute music, always falling into a great fright whenever the flute player began. Interestingly, this only occurred when he went out at night and never when he heard flute music during the day. The actual term *phobia* was first used by the Roman physician Celsus when he used the term *hydrophobia* (a fear of water) to describe someone that appeared to have a fear of water due to having rabies. The actual word 'phobia' is also derived from Greek from the god Phobos who was a great warrior and whose name literally means 'fear'.

Conceptions of madness from antiquity onwards

Little is documented in ancient texts about how people with mental disorders were treated in antiquity. In fact, people in many parts of the world did not differentiate between their physical and mental experiences and so the idea of a 'mental' disorder would have been completely alien to them (Wing, 1978). The earliest texts are from myths and religious stories and though they do mention people who lived with misery and fear, in general they were concerned with madness in a much more supernatural way, with the presumed cause of strange behaviour being possession by evil spirits or some other divine influence (Stone, 1998). They used the term 'madness' in a generic way that meant 'rage' or 'loss of one's mind' and this was usually identified by bizarre speech or behaviour in the sufferer. Ancient Babylonian and Mesopotamian texts attribute madness and strange behaviour to the malign influence of evil spirits. The Hebrews and other ancient peoples attributed diseases including madness to divine punishment for disobedience of god's laws (Pietikainen, 2015).

Even less can be derived from other civilisations, for example, in China from ancient times up until the mid-nineteenth century madness was not interpreted as a distinct illness and it did not seem to have become the focus of sustained medical attention or reflection, therefore there is little in the form of a written record (Scull, 2015). However, the relationship between human emotions and illness in Chinese writings goes as far back as the first century BC with the Inner Cannon of the Yellow Emperor and there were medical cases of emotional therapy from the late medieval period onwards (Chiang, 2014). With Western intervention into the far east came medical missionaries who brought with them the Western concepts of health and illness (Chen, 2003). The early Western investigations in to mental health in China led some to question whether mental illness actually existed in China, while others argued that it did but it's character was very different from that of its Western counterparts (ibid.). Madness was thought, as with other forms of ill-health, to derive from disharmony in bodily functions such as breathing, digestion and temperature regulation (Scull, 2015) and in this mind-body holism emotional disorders were thought to be closely associated with physical dysfunction, therefore, with such a view there was thought to be no need for a separate discipline of psychiatry (Chen, 2003). Madness in pre-modern China was more usually conceptualised as emotional disturbance and/or wild behaviour and treatments depended on the supposed cause – if it was thought to be due to natural environmental causes then treatments included herbal remedies, acupuncture and massage; if thought to be due to demonic attack then, just as was the case in the West the response to such a perceived demonic attack was to turn to exorcism (ibid.).

The great change in conceptions of madness in the Western world occurred during the Greek classical era with the development of Hippocratic medicine. The great philosophical shift was away from supernatural explanations of the world and illness towards rational explanations of phenomena that specifically looked for causes of illness within the human body. As part of this development in thought processes the brain began to be seen as a centre of mental activity. At Hippocratic medicine's core was the claim that the body was a system of interrelated elements. There were four of these and they were called the humours or fluids: blood (*haima*, which makes the body hot and wet); phlegm (*phlegma*, which makes the body cold and wet); black bile (*melan chole*, which makes the body cold and dry); and yellow bile (*chole*, which makes the body hot and dry) (Stone, 1998). Both mental and physical health depended on the balance between these bodily fluids. Madness was caused by a state of humeral imbalance. Melancholy, whose distinct features were sadness, fear and despair does, to a certain extent, resemble our modern conception of depression but it also referred to states of paranoia and to a type of catatonic stupor so it would be unwise to draw too close a parallel between the two. Melancholy was believed to be caused by an excess of black bile, whereas mania was caused by either an excess of phlegm or yellow bile. Those people with an excess of phlegm were thought to be quiet whereas those with an excess of yellow bile were thought to be frenzied and mischievous.

Though little is known about the treatments of mental distress in the ancient world we know from the writings of physicians, such as Galen, that the treatment of mania and melancholy was aimed at restoring a balance between the four humours and this included making patients sweat, vomit or suffer from diarrhoea to purge the excess of a particular humour. Considering how harsh life was for most people in antiquity some physicians held remarkably progressive views on treating those deemed 'mad'. Asclepiades (124–40 BCE) was possibly the first physician to differentiate between delusions (seeing an object but perceiving it as something else) and hallucinations (hearing or seeing things that others cannot hear or see) and he advocated a humane approach to the treatment of the mentally ill (ibid.). He treated the manic and melancholic with baths, massage, exercise, music therapy and a healthy diet and it has been noted that in the history of treating the mentally ill his approach was incredibly forward thinking for the time (Stone, 1998; Pietikainen, 2015). Soranus, a Greek physician from Ephesus, also believed in caring for rather than controlling the mentally ill. However, there were other far less enlightened figures though, such as Celsus, who recommended starving, chaining and whipping the mentally ill (Stone, 1998).

After the fall of the Western part of the Roman Empire in the fifth century Western thought was dominated by Christianity and a return to a supernatural world view and an end to Greek rationalism (Scull, 2015). In Europe during the period often described as the 'dark ages', which roughly covers the period from the sixth to the fourteenth centuries, the predominant Christian view was that human ailments both physical and mental were a consequence of man's fall from grace often resulting in demonic possession. The 'cure' for these ailments was often exorcism, prayer or visiting healing shrines. The Greek rationalist view, especially the medical writings of Galen, did survive however, in part because the eastern roman empire at Constantinople adopted Greek as the language of administration ensuring Greek medicine endured (ibid.) and, via an heretical Christian sect the Nestorians that found their way to Persia and, via this route, into Islamic medicine (Stone, 1998). With Islam's expansion into the west, especially the Iberian peninsula and Christian crusades into the Arab world, such contact between Islam and Christianity brought Galenic medicine back into western Europe – thought to be from the eleventh century onwards.

Through much of the period discussed above very few people were literate so little is known of the treatments of people with mental health problems (Scull, 2015). Anxiety disorders present a particular problem because, even after more medical treatises do start to appear from the sixteenth century onwards (e.g. Robert Burton's

The Anatomy of Melancholy of 1621), there is still no conception of particular anxiety disorders or attempts to differentiate anxiety from madness in general, or more specifically, unhappiness. In fact, Burton himself stated that fear and sorrow are the true characters of melancholy. Interestingly Burton had read some of the Arab texts that had rescued Galenic medicine from obscurity as can be seen by the fact that he cited the ninth century Egyptian Jewish physician Isaac Judaeus extensively (Pietikainen, 2015).

Furthermore, in fifteenth and sixteenth century Europe religious explanations for mental disorders and symptoms still had a significant influence. Thus, of over 2000 patients that the English clergyman and physician Richard Napier treated between 1597 and 1634, almost 300 of them were described as suffering from religious anxiety (ibid.). This often took the form of doubts about salvation and attempted cures often combined a mixture of magic, religion and science. Napier himself used, among other cures for mental illness, prayer, bleeding, purging, magic and astrology (see Figure 1.1).

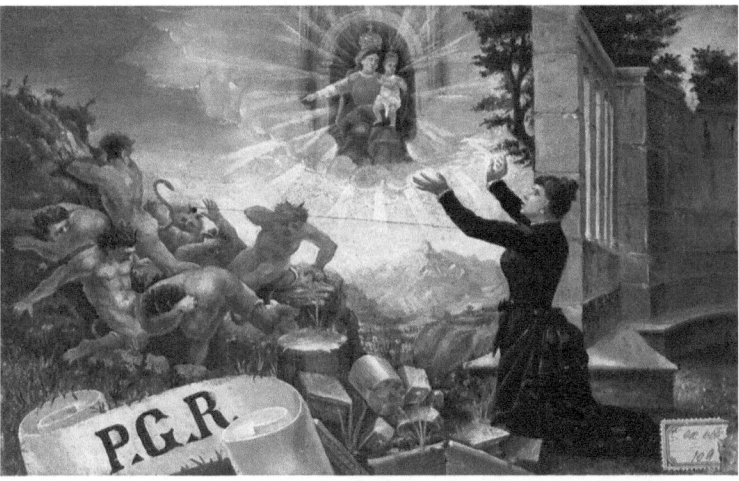

Figure 1.1 A woman expressing thanks to the Madonna del Parto for cure of insanity in the form of expelled devils. Oil painting. Sansovino, Iacopo, 1486–1570. Madonna del parto. (Wellcome Collection).

Gradually during the seventeenth century in northern Europe, as science and philosophy developed alongside trade and the growth of towns, societies also became more secular and less interested in the supernatural. This is important because, at this point, mental health problems again become perceived as illnesses primarily caused by biological or social causes and not as a result of demonic or other supernatural forces. As a consequence of this, magic amulets, prayers and exorcisms to cast out demons were no longer seen as sensible treatments for such ailments. Furthermore, mental illnesses came to be seen as the province of physicians and not priests or other practitioners of fantastical cures (Scull, 2015). However, one should be cautious when trying to describe the changes in concepts of madness and their associated treatments through history as wholly liberalist and evolutionist (Sedgwick, 1987). This approach views the past as barbarous and the present as the apex of enlightened treatment (ibid.) whereas currently, in some parts of the world, people hold very unenlightened views of mental health conditions and support and treatment is scarce. Even in the most wealthy countries, it would be extremely complacent to describe services as anywhere near perfect. In fact Sedgwick (ibid.) argued persuasively that one can see a constancy in some medical practices from antiquity up to modernity with the main innovations being not in treatments but in techniques. He cites the change from shocking a person by ducking them in cold water to shocking them with electricity and the change from trepanning to psychosurgery (rarely used now) as examples – indeed the confinement and restraint of people is something that has continued from antiquity up until the present day throughout the world.

The seventeenth century saw advances in human anatomy and physiology that had far reaching consequences for conceptions of emotional disorders. It was in the 1670s that the British physician Thomas Willis studied the human brain and nervous system and, based on his studies, argued that the nerves were the cause of many disorders including emotional disorders such as *hysteria*. Hysteria had long been seen as a purely female disorder caused by the movement of the womb within a woman's body. Now it was argued that it wasn't the womb but 'nerves' that caused emotional disorders and, equally importantly, that they could affect men as well as women (Showalter, 1997).

Up until this time hysteria, consisting as it did of a vast array of nonspecific emotional and physical symptoms, including lowness of spirits, exhaustion, paralyses and various aches and pains, was not something people wanted to be diagnosed with. An associated disorder *hypochondria* was thought to affect men in similar ways; this is not the modern conception of hypochondria but was so called because it was thought to originate in the hypochondrium; the upper abdomen (Scull, 2015). At this time hysteria was seen as an emotional disorder that had physical causes; later its character changed and it was then seen as a mental health issue that manifested itself in an array of physical symptoms usually neurological in character such as numbness, blindness or paralysis. One of the most famous people to exhibit such symptoms was Adolf Hitler who suddenly became blind while fighting in the trenches in World War I – it was recognised that his blindness was hysterical in origin and he was successfully treated with psychological interventions in a Pomeranian nerve clinic in 1918 (Achtler, 2008). It has been noted (Showalter, 1997) that hysteria is a disorder that has changed its character on numerous occasions throughout history by mimicking culturally permissible expressions of distress.

Back in the eighteenth century the low opinion of nervous disorders was challenged when George Cheyne published in 1733 *A Treatise of Nervous Diseases of all Kinds*, interestingly its main title was the 'English malady'. In this book he managed to change the perception of nervous diseases by arguing that they weren't imaginary disorders better attributed to human weakness but were real and had a physical cause, specifically the recently discovered nerves. Furthermore, he also argued they were diseases caused by civilisation and therefore the more civilised a society was it followed that its most civilised citizens would be the ones most prone to such nervous diseases. This, of course, played to the vanity of certain types of people, especially those in the higher echelons of English society who wished to be perceived as highly refined.

Specific anxiety disorders

Social anxiety disorder

During the seventeenth and eighteenth centuries in Europe great advances were made in philosophy and science during an era that is known as the Enlightenment. Political changes also took place as absolutist monarchies had to relinquish some powers to their parliaments and a small number of wealthy people benefitted from these first small democratic steps. However, wielding power, making important decisions concerning domestic and international relations and being seen doing these things by arguing for political positions involves a considerable amount of public speaking. This is something that does not always sit easily with those that ascend to such high office. An example of one such individual is John Stuart, third Earl of Bute (1713–1792). Bute became British prime minister and served from 1762 to 1763 but, like many people who desire the limelight in one form or another, he found it intensely anxiety provoking when thrust into it (Davidson, 2011). He was described as deeply insecure, cold and distant and he found it difficult to mix in society. It would appear, therefore, that primarily he suffered from social anxiety disorder. His natural shyness was probably compounded by the fact that he knew that he was not liked by many of his political associates as he had been the 'finishing tutor' to the future king, King George III, and thus was perceived to have become prime minister due only to his political connections. He also became the first Scottish prime minister only 17 years after the second Jacobite rebellion had attempted to return the Scottish Stuarts to the British throne, which would also have made many distrustful of him.

Being prime minister requires attendance at many public engagements which are also often accompanied by public speaking; for a person with social anxiety disorder, such as Bute, these public performance situations would be highly anxiety provoking. As is often the case, his increasing anxiety level then triggered a depressive episode and his increasing level of illness was a significant contributing factor to his resigning as prime minister within a year (ibid.). During his time in office he took copious amounts of hemlock, a plant that can be used as a sedative if taken in small enough doses (though fatal in large doses) with little effect. It appears that, as often occurs with people with social anxiety disorder, his anxieties only lessened when he avoided those situations that provoked his anxiety and it was noted that both his anxiety and his mood improved after leaving office.

Social anxiety disorder was first categorised as a phobia in the American Diagnostic and Statistical Manual (DSM-III) in 1980 and at that time was described as *social phobia*. As stated earlier it is one of the most common anxiety disorders. What social anxiety disorder is *not,* is excessive shyness – it is not the case that psychiatrists have taken a common personality trait such as shyness and transformed it into a mental health condition. Many people who are shy do not experience the negative emotions and feelings that accompany social anxiety disorder. They live a normal life, and do not view shyness as a negative trait. On the flip side, it isn't the case that people with social anxiety disorder are necessarily shy. People with social anxiety disorder endure significant anxiety on a daily basis and view the condition extremely negatively whereas some people may view their shyness as a positive quality.

As we will see, many people who would be perceived to be extroverts, or have chosen careers that involve a significant amount of public performance, have suffered from social anxiety and this has seriously affected their ability to pursue the career of their choice. One such career choice is politics. Only three years after the third Earl of Bute left office, the next but one British prime minister was Charles Watson-Wentworth, the second Marquess of Rockingham, who in his first stint as prime minister lasted only three months due to cabinet conflict. He found public speaking very distressing and at times was described as 'tongue-tied' while trying to speak in parliament and, like Bute before him, sought his own medicinal remedy for his anxiety – in his case he sometimes drank Madeira before speaking and had his physician bleed him afterwards (bleeding was then seen as a treatment for almost any physical ailment) (ibid.). His second stint as prime minister was 16 years later and, unfortunately, only lasted 14 weeks as he died during the influenza epidemic of 1782.

Despite the amount of public scrutiny politicians have always been under (admittedly much more in the modern age, though relatively speaking they always have been) it is interesting how many have experienced a considerable amount of social anxiety disorder. It has been estimated (Davidson et al., 2006) that it is highly likely that three of the first 37 US presidents had social anxiety disorder, namely, Thomas Jefferson, Ulysses Grant and Calvin Coolidge. Though in the case of Coolidge, when he first became president in

1923, he instituted regular press conferences and convened meetings and engaged with members of Congress which is not indicative of social anxiety disorder. He actually became much more withdrawn and less interested in public speaking after the sudden death of his son Calvin Jr in July 1924 just after he had been re-elected, and some have argued (Gilbert, 2003) that he was actually clinically depressed.

The words of the pioneering American nurse Clara Barton (1821–1912) highlight that social anxiety often occurs from an early age when she wrote in her memoirs: 'I had grown even more timid, shrinking and sensitive in the presence of others; absurdly careful and methodical for a child' (Barton, 1907). Her parents' combustible relationship, her mother's strange behaviour and having an older sister who was so mentally unwell that she was kept in a locked room at home seems to have adversely affected her. She became less anxious after caring for her brother for two years after he injured himself in a fall (ibid.). This she did from the age of 11 and it had such a profound effect on her that she became a nurse in her adulthood when the American Civil War broke out, at which time she earned the nick name 'angel of the battlefield'. In 1881 she founded the American Red Cross. Throughout her adult life she had to give many speeches and, despite hating public speaking, she forced herself to do it. She also suffered from periodic depressive episodes, describing them as like being followed by 'thin black snakes'; episodes that only lifted when she threw herself into another work project.

Another sufferer of social phobia who had to try his best to deal with increasing public interest was Orville Wright (1871–1948), famed for the first free, controlled flight of a power-driven aeroplane. This first flight was in 1903 and it wouldn't be until 1908 that he and his brother became famous by demonstrating how well a later version of their flying machine worked. It was commented that Orville, like many people with a social phobia, was very quiet and reticent to speak in public but was much more relaxed and forthcoming at home among his family where he obviously did not fear any negative judgemental reactions. It is ironic that someone brave enough to be one of the first humans to take to the skies in what was an extremely rudimentary, flimsy and, therefore, dangerous flying machine had such a fear of public speaking. He let his brother, Wilbur, be the public face of their business until Wilbur died in 1912 at the age of 45 of typhoid. There is no record of him ever receiving any form of treatment for his social phobia but that was not uncommon in the first half of the twentieth century.

As previously mentioned, social phobia first became recognised as a disorder in 1980 and, as with any disorder, official recognition encouraged clinicians to be more comfortable diagnosing it and so the number of those diagnosed grew significantly. It is estimated that there are 15 million people with social anxiety disorder in America alone (www.adaa.org/understanding-anxiety/social-anxiety-disorder). Examples of people who have talked about their social anxiety disorder include the singer Donny Osmond – like many people who have social anxiety disorder he noticed his anxiety from an early age but tried to ignore it and carry on with his public performing until he was no longer able to do so. He has described how he became paralysed with fear while performing in *Joseph and the Amazing Technicolour Dreamcoat*. Like many people he has been treated with a combination of antidepressants and a therapy called cognitive behavioural therapy (CBT) that have helped him to control his anxious thoughts and feelings. CBT has been researched extensively and has been shown to be one of the most effective talking treatments for depression and anxiety disorders (Clark, 1999). Many studies also recommend a combination of both CBT and antidepressants (Craske & Stein, 2016).

The central tenet of CBT is that how we think affects how we feel and this in turn affects how we behave, this is also the interpretation or meaning that people give to the experiences that influence their emotional and behavioural reactions (Rachman, 1999). Often people interpret events to be far more threatening than they are and this provokes negative emotions such as anxiety and depression. For example, people who experience panic disorder often misinterpret a symptom of anxiety, such as palpitations, as a sign of an impending heart attack and this increases their anxiety even further as they fear they are about to die (Clark, 1999).

CBT focusses on these faulty interpretations of events and tries to help people develop a more balanced interpretation of them. It also tries to identify what people do to try to 'save' themselves when they are in a state of fear. For example, a person with social anxiety will avoid a feared situation such as public speaking because they

will have a mental picture of themselves performing badly, probably stammering, their mind going blank, maybe even going red and
sweating profusely. They will then picture the audience reaction as
wholly negative; for example, people laughing at them, pointing at
them and maybe even walking out of the room in anger. The fact
that they avoid these situations means they never test out these
negative predictions and so their belief in them is always very strong,
often 100 per cent.

Having identified these negative thoughts and predictions, the CBT
therapist, in collaboration with the client, can devise what are called
'behavioural experiments' – in these various forms of the feared situation are gradually developed. In social phobia, identifying the person's
safety behaviours is vital. For example, people who fear social situations try to get them over with quickly by talking rapidly. A therapist
addressing this behaviour will encourage the person to talk slowly,
when in a social situation, possibly even introduce a boring subject
on purpose and then observe the reaction of people around them.
Usually people discover that their feared outcome that people would
look bored or reject them in some manner doesn't occur (ibid.) and
this, and further behavioural experiments, overtime undermines the
strength of their belief that social situations are personally threatening.

It is interesting that so many people who can best be described
as public entertainers, such as actors and singers, also suffer from
social anxiety. This is testament to the willpower and determination
of people to follow their dreams despite the fact that it may entail
doing something that provokes such fear for them. Other examples
of people who have talked openly of their social anxiety include the
actor Kim Basinger, the singers Carly Simon and Barbara Streisand
and the American football player Ricky Williams. Basinger has talked
openly about her anxiety and how she has lived with it all her life.
In the film *Panic: A Film About Coping* she talked about how being
asked to read out loud in front of the rest of her classmates made her
incredibly anxious to the point that she dreaded going to school.
This led to her having panic attacks in her twenties. This is also very
common with anxiety disorders, where people often have more than
one anxiety disorder; in fact it got so bad for her that at one stage she
remained in her house for months, too fearful to go out. Even having
people round to her home began to make her anxious.

Streisand has spoken about how she doesn't remember her good reviews but the negative ones stay in her mind. This is very typical of social anxiety disorder, as people with it discount any complements or praise they receive – especially if received from a friend or a loved one, as they will think that the person offering praise has to do so because of their close relationship. However, negative comments act like a lightning bolt hitting right to the core of the person, as they seem to add further proof to the individual's low opinion of themselves. Like Donny Osmond, Streisand has used both medication and therapy to treat her anxiety, indeed it has been reported that they have both actually used the same therapist.

Obsessive compulsive disorder

Obsessive Compulsive Disorder (OCD) can be described as anxiety expressed as ritual. It is characterised by recurrent obsessions including intrusive thoughts, images and impulses and/or compulsions which include compelling repetitive behaviours or mental acts intended to put right or neutralise the obsession (Westbrook et al., 2008). For these thoughts and behaviours to be seen as a disorder they have to be recurrent and persistent and the person, at some point, has to recognise that the obsessions/compulsions are excessive and unreasonable and that they are causing them distress.

The most common obsessional fears include: fears of contamination; fears that they will make a mistake or forget to do something important such as turn a gas tap off, unplug the iron or leave a door unlocked; fears of behaving inappropriately such as shouting out swear words in church or another inappropriate place; being violent to loved ones or behaving in a sexually inappropriate manner; and an over concern with orderliness or perfection (ibid.). To counter these obsessions, people develop compulsive behaviours such as rituals that they use to reassure themselves that the unwelcome, intrusive thoughts won't occur. For example, people with a fear that they will leave a gas tap on will ritually turn it on and off usually a specific number of times 'just to make sure' that it is turned off. Unfortunately, the more people think about the issue the more anxious they become and the number of times that they have to enact the ritual to reassure themselves often increases. These themes seem to be consistent across cultures – a study in India noted that the most common themes were concerned with issues such as dirt and contamination, orderliness, sex and religion, exactly the same as those described by Western patients (Toates & Coschung-Toates, 2005).

Intrusive thoughts also have a long history, with mentions of them in early Buddhist writings in the fifth century BC (ibid.). Like other anxiety disorders, one of the earliest Western descriptions of OCD was by Robert Burton in his *The Anatomy of Melancholy* (1621) in which he described a case of an individual that was worried about speaking something 'indecent' while at a sermon. The French psychiatrist Pierre Janet working in the late nineteenth and early twentieth century was one of the first to study obsessions in great detail, especially in his work *Lés Obsessions et la Psychasthénie* (Obsessions and Psychasthenia) .

An early example of an individual with OCD is the theologian Martin Luther (1483–1546); he was one of the leading figures in the Reformation, which was an attempt to reform the Catholic Church but which led to a schism within it. In 1516 the Roman Catholic Church sent a papal commissioner to Germany to sell indulgences to raise money to rebuild St Peter's Basilica in Rome. Indulgences were a way of reducing the penance required for a sin while alive, or the temporal punishment one would experience in purgatory after death. Essentially they were an 'insurance policy' against the size of one's punishment for one's indiscretions sold with the authority of the Pope.

Luther rejected the view that freedom from God's punishment could be paid for with money and he insisted the Pope had no authority over purgatory. This, and other differences with the prevailing views of the Church, brought him into direct conflict with the Pope and resulted in his eventual excommunication from the Church in 1521. It's generally accepted that Luther experienced persistent intrusive thoughts of a blasphemous nature. He believed also that his attempts to repent for his lustful and blasphemous thoughts by prayer failed as these thoughts returned. His form of OCD is called *scrupulosity*, which is characterised by persistent, irrational, unwanted beliefs and thoughts about not being devout or moral enough, despite all evidence to the contrary. Luther tried to deal with his unwanted thoughts by suppressing them. This is a very common way in which people with OCD try to deal with distressing intrusive thoughts. The problem with trying to supress thoughts is that the more a person tries not to think of something, the more they do think of it so, it is never successful.

John Bunyan (1628–1688), the author of *The Pilgrim's Progress*, was another sufferer of scrupulosity. He had become a nonconformist preacher in the period of the English Civil War but, after the restoration of the monarchy in 1660, such religious freedoms were curtailed. In 1661 he was charged with attending a religious gathering at a venue other than his parish church. He was sentenced to three months in prison and had to agree to desist from preaching, this he refused to do and he eventually served 12 years in prison! He spoke at length in his spiritual autobiography *Grace Abounding to the Chief of Sinners* (1666) about his intrusive thoughts in which he worried that rather than praise God he would utter blasphemous accusations against him (ibid.). Rather than try to suppress these thoughts Bunyan actually physically restrained himself by putting his hand under his chin to keep his mouth shut (Veale & Wilson, 2009). It's not reported how successful this strategy was though, even if it worked in the very short term, it is unlikely that one could go about one's business on a daily basis while holding one's mouth shut.

Intrusive religious thoughts aren't the only symptoms of OCD. Dr Samuel Johnson (1709–1784) who was a poet, essayist, biographer and the man credited with compiling the most comprehensive dictionary of the English Language at the time (it took him nine years working single-handedly and he finished it in 1755), was also prone to a number of strange mannerisms. It has been argued, with good evidence, that his odd gestures and tics should confer on him a diagnosis of Tourette's syndrome; his obituarist, Thomas Tyrer, called him a 'convulsionary' (Porter, 1985). These strange movements were so noticeable that when the artist Hogarth first saw Johnson he thought he had a learning disability (in the language of the time he stated he thought Johnson was an 'ideot'). Though it is highly likely that he did suffer from Tourette's syndrome it also seems likely he suffered from OCD. He was observed to touch every post he passed as he walked along the street, and if he missed one he would go back to ensure he touched it, he had a habit of rubbing pieces of orange peel together and he engaged in an elaborate ritual when crossing over the threshold of any doorway. He would whirl and twist to perform various gesticulations then when finished would suddenly, with an extensive stride, cross the threshold. This he would do not just on entering a building but also at any subsequent doorway. Boswell, in his biography entitled *Life of Samuel Johnson,* described his 'anxious care' and 'superstitious habit' at doorways where he would also count the number of steps he took in his approach to a doorway. He had so many of these different ruminations and rituals that Porter has described Johnson as 'riddled with private phobias and grotesque compulsions' (ibid., p. 68).

Alongside such rituals Johnson also exhibited other symptoms of anxiety, such as a tendency to worry a lot; indeed he worried about his mental health to such a degree that a friend, Mrs Thrale, stated that 'his over-anxious care to retain without blemish the perfect sanity of his mind, contributed much to disturb it' (quoted in Porter, 1985, p. 67). This is what would now be called a meta-worry – to worry about how much you are worrying is also very common to many anxiety disorders and is treated today by cognitive therapy. It is also clear that Johnson's early life contributed to his anxiety in adulthood, he was half-blind in his left eye and half-deaf in his left ear due to scrofula (an infection of the lymph nodes usually caused by tuberculosis) as a child and he was large and clumsy. When he went to the University of Oxford he was forced to leave due to a lack of funds. He was often short of funds and constantly found life to be a disappointment; all of these life stressors would have added to his anxieties and made it difficult for him to escape them.

For someone else wracked by a whole range of intrusive ruminations and associated compulsive rituals we need look no further than the famous Danish writer Hans Christian Andersen (1805–1875). He had intrusive thoughts that, for example, what he had eaten would poison him, that he would be returned to poverty, while out he would incessantly worry he had forgotten to lock his front door, he would worry he had mixed up the envelopes when sending letters and, among other ruminations, he would worry he had paid the wrong amount of money in shops. He felt compelled to act on his intrusive thoughts, for example, he continually got up at night to check he had extinguished his candle, he carried a rope in his trunk in case of a fire so that he could descend from a window, and kept a note by his bedside that roughly translated as 'I'm only sleeping' due to his fear of being buried alive (he also asked a friend to cut one of his arteries before sealing his coffin just to be certain he was dead). Luckily, like Johnson before him, he wrote extensively about his obsessive thoughts. This gave future generations a glimpse into how their thoughts made them so anxious and could affect their behaviour in their day-to-day lives. Johnson wrote many letters and kept a diary and Andersen wrote an autobiography in which he detailed his obsessions. Like other figures from before the twentieth century treatments were rarely sought – Samuel Johnson, like many others across the ages, prayed to God for salvation from his intrusive thoughts and even went as far as visiting a condemned man to ask him to make a plea on his behalf when he reached the other side (Toates & Coschung-Toates, 2005).

One of the most famous figures with OCD is the engineer, industrialist, aviation pioneer, film producer and director Howard Hughes (1905–1976). He was himself the subject of a successful film called *The Aviator* in which he was played by Leonardo DiCaprio, an actor who has stated that he has mild-to-moderate OCD and used his insight into the condition to help him in the role of Hughes. Hughes' mother was highly overprotective and was constantly worrying and monitoring his physical and emotional well-being. He was only 16 when she died at the age of 39 from complications of an ectopic pregnancy, his father died of a heart attack only two years later. Losing both parents at such a young age would only have compounded the worries about his own health that his mother had been instilling in him from very early on.

Hughes was socially anxious and described as always a little eccentric. Despite this, he enjoyed a highly successful business career in engineering, real estate investments and produced a number of successful films. He was also passionate about aviation and was involved in all aspects of the process from design to actually flying various models of aeroplanes. Unfortunately, he was involved in two near fatal aeroplane crashes, one in 1943 and one in 1946; the second crash was in the Beverly Hills neighbourhood of Los Angeles. It appears that his eccentricities began in earnest after he recovered from his injuries from the crash (ibid.). It is thought that Hughes had developed a condition called *allodynia* after the aeroplane crashes. This is a complex condition that leaves the sufferer experiencing a massively increased pain response to stimuli that would not usually cause pain. In Hughes' case, after the crash, he found it incredibly painful to wear clothes and so sat around for four months watching movies while wearing nothing but a napkin covering his genitals. Over time he also became addicted to the opiate-based painkiller, codeine. Hughes, always regarded as eccentric, now became even more bizarre in his behaviour; he started to become paranoid and focussed on seeing people as laden in germs (ibid.). He retreated further from public life and spent most of the last ten years of his life living in penthouse suites in hotels, obsessed with germs and contamination. He hardly ever washed or cut his hair or toenails. He ate very little and when he died he was suffering from malnutrition, weighing only 41 kg (90 lbs); he was 6ft 4in. in height.

It is clear that his status as a billionaire able to surround himself with people who would do whatever he paid them to do made Hughes very vulnerable to his increasing obsessions and isolation. Any 'ordinary' individual who had exhibited such extreme obsessional behaviour and self-neglect would have been encouraged, or maybe even forced, to accept medical or mental health treatment. Hughes, being so rich, was perceived as 'eccentric' and was indulged, very much to his detriment.

Thirty years earlier a similar fate had met the famous inventor Nikola Tesla, he too suffered from OCD and in his final years lived off Nabisco crackers and milk. Furthermore, he also lived in hotels and died in one alone and emaciated just like Hughes. Tesla was also an inventor and developed a motor that ran on alternating current. He had a fear of germs and was repulsed by pearls! Paradoxically, in later life he became a columbiphile, a person who loves pigeons, and he would feed them daily, allowing many to sit on parts of his body (Pickover, 1999). Tesla had numerous rituals to contain his anxiety, for example, he had to have 18 napkins at his table when he ate and many other things had to come in numbers divisible by three.

When asked about this he could give no rational explanation. His intelligence, public profile and, at times, wealth meant that Tesla, like Hughes, garnered the label 'eccentric' rather than 'mentally ill'. Any ordinary person that behaved in such strange ways would have been treated differently and not given such a wide degree of latitude in their behaviour. It's clear that money and power are a double-edged sword – on the one hand they allow an individual an awful lot more freedom in how they behave (they can certainly get away with a lot more than the average person without being subject to a response from agencies such as the police or mental health services) while, on the other hand, they are sometimes not given the help they need and are vulnerable to being indulged in their self-destructive behaviour by family, friends or by paid employees that are all too willing to indulge them in their self-destructive behaviour if the money's good enough.

A fear of contamination and germs is very common with OCD and a number of famous people suffer with this. The film actor Megan Fox has said that the phobia means she won't use public toilets or restaurant silverware. In a similar vein the actor Cameron Diaz has admitted that her fear of catching germs from doorknobs means she opens doors with her elbows and cleans the doors at her home so often that the paint was cleaned off them. Both actors have been successful in controlling their compulsions so that they have not become a hindrance to their successful careers. Fox has said that the birth of her first child led to a reduction in her obsessive thoughts and compulsive behaviours. Other famous sufferers of the disorder include: the former footballer David Beckham, who has an issue with pairing items and ordering things by colour or type; and the actor and singer Billy Bob Thornton, who associates people with certain numbers and says that that means he is constantly doing mathematics in his head, which he can find exhausting.

In their book on OCD (Toates & Coschung-Toates, 2005) Dr Frederick Toates, a professor at the Open University and sufferer of OCD himself, discusses the three main ways in which OCD is treated. These are: behavioural therapy, especially repeated exposure to the feared situation; techniques to reshape the person's thinking, such as cognitive therapy; and medication. In clinical practice in the

UK, however, the three are usually used in combination. Behavioural therapy is difficult to use with patients who have no overt ritualistic behaviours. The basic behavioural technique is exposure and response prevention (ERP). In ERP the person with OCD is encouraged to 'expose' themselves to the feared situation without engaging in their usual safety behaviours, for example, touching door handles without washing one's hands immediately afterwards. Over time the degree of anxiety associated with the 'contamination' reduces as the person realises that nothing bad has happened to them as a consequence of their activity. People often find such approaches challenging and pure behavioural approaches tend to have a high refusal or early drop-out rate (Salkovskis & Kirk, 1999). For that reason, behavioural and cognitive components are often combined.

The cognitive component of therapy focusses on challenging unhelpful beliefs such as 'if I think it, it will happen', and the individual's belief that they will be responsible for harm to themselves or others if they fail to take action to prevent the harm from occurring. The aim of therapy is to help the person conclude that obsessional thoughts are irrelevant to further action (ibid.). Intrusive thoughts can be distressing and, early on in the therapy sessions, the therapist tries to normalise them by discussing how common they are and how in some circumstances they can be helpful, for example, when they occur in moderation they may be a way of thinking about potential dangers and planning to avoid them or deciding on what to do if they occur. A key characteristic of intrusive thoughts is their unplanned spontaneous nature, therefore, in therapy it is useful to ask the individual questions such as: What it would be like if you had no intrusive thoughts and had to decide on your next thought?; How would you choose what to think and would such a process be boring?

Medication is often used in combination with therapeutic interventions. Sometimes it may be the only treatment, as some people are not psychologically-minded and are unable or unwilling to participate in a talking therapy. Of course, in some parts of the world talking therapies are not available. The most commonly used medication is antidepressants and, of those available, the category of Selective Serotonin Reuptake Inhibitors (SSRIs) has the best evidence base for use with OCD (NICE, 2005). There are a number of these drugs that have a licence for treating OCD. Clinical evidence suggests that, even after the patient has responded and appears to be in remission, they should continue the medication for at least 12 months to avoid relapse and allow for further improvements. After this time the treating clinician should review the need for the medication with the patient and consider its gradual withdrawal.

Panic disorder

As was described earlier in the chapter, a panic attack is defined as a 'sudden episode of intense fear and panic'. What makes them particularly unsettling for the sufferer is that they tend to occur suddenly, without warning and often for no discernible reason (Clark, 1999). Its subtitle in the WHO diagnostic manual, the ICD-10, is 'episodic paroxysmal anxiety' which succinctly describes its true nature. Panic attacks are common to many mental health conditions. They are often seen in people who have agoraphobia, they are common to people who have depression and often occur in people who are suffering from other anxiety disorders. Common symptoms include: palpitations, pounding heart, sweating, shaking, chest pain, nausea, a churning stomach, feeling light headed, a fear of dying, and losing control or going mad. For a person to be diagnosed with panic disorder they have to experience at least four of the main symptoms listed above, the attacks have to reach a crescendo within a few minutes and last at least some minutes (WHO, 1993). They also have to be recurrent. Often when people have had a panic attack they worry about having further attacks, this has been described as the 'cycle of fear'. The frequency of panic attacks varies widely among sufferers from daily to less than monthly. Given the number of physical symptoms associated with panic attacks it is no surprise that there is an increased risk of developing panic disorder for sufferers of several physical conditions including cardiovascular disorders, chronic obstructive pulmonary disease (COPD) and asthma. Women are two- to three-times more likely to develop panic disorder than men.

Deriving its name from the ancient Greek woodland god Pan (a half man half goat, horned creature who liked to spread fear by harassing nymphs) 'panic' was not originally thought of as being particularly distinct from terror or fear. Prior to the nineteenth century it was common for folk healers and physicians alike to treat each individual symptom as a separate medical complaint (Nardi, 2006). Often these physical symptoms were seen purely as arising from a physical cause, for example palpitations were seen as a disease of the heart. The first description of what we would recognise as panic disorder occurred in 1873 when Maurice Krishaber associated dizziness, tachycardia and restlessness to one neurocirculatory disease (ibid.).

The second half of the nineteenth century saw a greater identification of the fact that anxiety disorders were disorders in their own right and not just symptoms of depression. Freud's descriptions of anxiety neurosis include a description of anxiety attacks that are identical to the modern conception of panic disorder. An important part of Freud's description is that he separated anxiety neurosis from chronic anxiety states and described it as an acute anxiety attack (ibid.). However it was not until 1980 that *panic disorder* was fully described and recognised as a condition when it was included in the third edition of the DSM.

A number of factors have been identified that make panic disorder worse including alcohol misuse, caffeine, illicit drug misuse and smoking, especially from a young age. Though it has been found to run in families there is no established genetic link and a whole host of social factors, such as family coping styles and stressful family environments mean that the relationship between panic disorder and familial transmission is complex and not well understood (Linden, 2012).

As panic disorder has only been clearly identified and described relatively recently, there are no historical references to it. Furthermore, the fact that it often occurs alongside, or as a consequence of, other disorders means that it is not as easy to be sure if historic figures had panic disorder or experienced occasional panic attacks alongside, for example, a depressive illness. A good modern example of this is Kim Basinger; as discussed, she experienced social anxiety disorder and then developed panic disorder in her twenties.

Charlie Beljan, the American golfer, experienced such severe panic attacks while competing in a tournament in November 2012 at Disney World that he thought he was having a heart attack (which is a common fear for people experiencing panic attacks) and was taken in an ambulance to hospital. He returned to continue to compete in the tournament and actually won it. To date this remains his only PGA Tour win. When Beljan spoke about his panic disorder fellow golfer Bubba Watson disclosed that he, too, has experienced panic disorder and has attended hospitals three times believing there was something wrong with his heart. He also withdrew from the Northern Trust Open in Los Angeles in 2011 after suffering a panic attack during the tournament.

A number of famous people have spoken about their panic attacks and both Amanda Seyfried the actor and Ellie Goulding the singer have discussed how therapy has helped them. Goulding has described how CBT was beneficial in helping her to control her anxiety. Like Beljan, Goulding thought she was having a heart attack when she had her first panic attack and went to hospital she was that concerned. The British singer Adele has described experiencing numerous panic attacks on stage and this has led her to turn down some events such as the Glastonbury festival due to their size. Having to appear at a huge event also provoked a panic attack in the singer Missy Elliott who described it happening to her before she went on at half time during Super Bowl XLIX in 2015.

The American actor and writer Lena Dunham has stated that what has helped her to deal with her anxiety has been both medication and exercise. She challenged the image common in films of medication as making women 'hollowed out' versions of themselves but stated that they were, in fact, helpful and were part of the process of helping her get better. She has also been a strong advocate for exercise, stating that she was surprised just how much it helped her anxiety. A review of studies that evaluated the use of exercise in anxiety disorders (Ravindran & da Silva, 2013) found that several studies found exercise used to augment other treatments helped in both GAD and panic disorder. People exercising will benefit from the release of various chemicals within the brain including the neuropeptide endorphins that can induce a euphoria-like state and others that modulate stress reactivity. However, a biological explanation is only part of the reason for improvements related to increased levels of exercise. The physical act of exercising also distracts the person from their worrying thoughts, they also gain a sense of self-worth for actually doing something for themselves to improve their condition and if they start to feel physically fitter and notice positive changes to their physical condition (e.g. loss of excess body fat) this also raises their self-esteem and has a positive impact on their personal confidence.

As with other anxiety disorders the talking therapy with the best evidence base for use with panic disorder is CBT. In the cognitive model of panic the person with panic disorder is thought to have an enduring tendency to interpret a wide range of bodily sensations in a catastrophic way (Clark, 1999). For example, people often interpret their anxiety symptoms as a sign that they are having a heart attack. The bodily sensations that accompany a heart attack also normally occur when someone is anxious such as increased heart rate, feeling hot and flushed and becoming sweaty. The person misinterprets these as a sign of an impending physical or mental collapse. The therapist identifies these catastrophic interpretations then tries via questioning to help the patient derive non-catastrophic alternative explanations.

For example, if a person fears that they will have a heart attack if they exercise vigorously, as many celebrities discussed earlier did, then one of the goals of therapy is to help them understand that they are misinterpreting anxiety as a serious medical condition. Usually people who fear having a heart attack if they exercise avoid exercising and, whenever they notice an increase in their heart rate, they adopt safety behaviours such as sitting down. The therapist will encourage them to drop the safety behaviours and over subsequent weeks develop experiments that involve greater degrees of exercise all the time undermining the strength of their belief which will lead to a reduction in the emotional response provoked by that belief (ibid.). If patients do drop their safety behaviours, research suggests that the reduction in anxiety is much more significant than if they just focus on their interpretations of their bodily sensations. A number of studies have demonstrated the efficacy of CBT and it has been noted that the development of computer-based CBT packages has made it a much more accessible therapy (Craske & Stein, 2016).

Medication also has a role in treating panic disorder. Various classes of antidepressants have been seen to be equally effective; SSRIs, Tricyclic antidepressants (TCAs) and Mono Amine Oxidase Inhibitors (MAOIs) are the three different types that have all demonstrated their effectiveness in clinical trials (Linden, 2012). The choice of which to use is a clinical decision taking into account such factors as previous treatment response, tolerability and preference. A further important factor is risk, if the individual has suicidal thoughts then TCAs and MAOIs should be avoided as TCAs are highly toxic in overdose and MAOIs have dangerous interactions with a number of common foodstuffs. Medications should be used in conjunction with a talking therapy as the two combined have been found to be far more effective than either being used individually (Craske & Stein, 2016).

Post-traumatic Stress Disorder (PTSD)

PTSD can be described as a relatively new disorder in that it has only been officially recognised since it was added to the DSM-III by the American Psychiatric Association in 1980 (Turnbull, 2012). However, this only marks its official recognition as it has long been recognised that following exposure to traumatic events people may develop emotional and psychological difficulties. Prevalence rates for PTSD have been estimated to range from 0.3% to 6.1% in general populations globally, and 15.4% in conflict-affected populations (WHO, 2013). An early example of trauma associated with battle comes from the Greek philosopher and historian Herodotus who, in his epic account of the Greco-Persian wars, described a soldier at the Battle of Marathon who after witnessing the death of a fellow soldier next to him went totally blind despite being completely uninjured himself. The inference is that the blindness was an emotional reaction to the trauma he had experienced rather than derived from a physical cause.

Situations that can trigger PTSD in an individual include: being subject to a traumatic event that involved actual or threatened death or injury; a threat to the physical integrity of the person or others (such as sexual violence); and indirect exposure such as learning about the violent or accidental death or perpetration of sexual violence to a loved one. An example of such a shocking traumatic event occurred to Franklin Pierce (1804–1869), the fourteenth President of the United States, and it is suggested (Davidson et al., 2006) that in all likelihood he experienced PTSD after the traumatic death of his last surviving son, Benjamin, in a train crash. The child was killed and nearly decapitated, something seen by both Pierce and his wife who were also in the crash. The crash occurred only weeks after his election as president and its effects are thought to have contributed to his poor performance in office.

Given the amount of trauma people have endured throughout history and that the twentieth century included two cataclysmic world wars engulfing many millions of people it is surprising that it took so long for the disorder to be recognised, described and accepted. One of the main reasons it took so long was that the whole concept of external events having such a profound psycho-logical effect on an individual wasn't accepted by the medical profession until very recently (Trimble, 1985). In the nineteenth century the prevailing wisdom was still that traumatic shock was caused by physical damage to some part of the nervous system. It was thought that physical injuries to the head or spinal cord or cer-ebral haemorrhages were responsible for the psychological distress that people displayed (ibid.). This meant that even when soldiers did exhibit psychological distress during or after campaigns in the nineteenth century they were described in physical terms such as palpitations, debility, disordered action of the heart and rheumatism (Jones et al., 2003).

There is evidence that culture has an influence on how people express their distress as Jones et al. (2003) found when reviewing the medical files of British service personnel from 1854 onwards. They found that flashbacks, one of the key symptoms of PTSD, were conspicuous by their absence in the files of service personnel before World War I and were still rare during World Wars I and II. They argue that the development of the television age and the introduc-tion of the idea that one can cut back to a scene from the past has been a factor in shaping how people express distress.

An interest in the effects of trauma on people gained impetus dur-ing the First World War of 1914–1918. This was the first fully mod-ern war with the use of large-scale armaments and involving death and suffering on a truly industrial scale. In the first year of the war many soldiers began to present with symptoms of psychological dis-tress including amnesia, headaches, dizziness and tremors. In 1915 Charles Myers, a British psychologist, published an article in the

British medical journal, *The Lancet,* discussing the phenomenon – he used the term 'shell shock', a term that was being used commonly at the time and which attributed the psychological symptoms the soldiers presented with to the concussive effects of bomb blasts (Turnbull, 2012). Thinking in these terms, many physicians still believed that there was some hidden physical damage caused by the bomb blasts that caused the psychological distress. Others such as Myers noted, however, that some of the soldiers exhibited these symptoms without coming under fire, inferring that shell shock was not a result of physical damage caused by bomb blasts.

The British Army also began to distinguish between those soldiers who seemed to be experiencing an emotional breakdown after combat and those who had not been in combat prior to their symptoms occurring. They distinguished between them by pre-fixing a '*W*' to the casualty report of those that had been in action denoting 'wounded', whereas for those that exhibited such symptoms but had not been in action, their casualty report was prefixed with an '*S*' for 'sick'. Those that received the '*S*' were denied a wound stripe and in some cases their war pension too (ibid.). The British Army estimated that only 4–10 per cent of shell shock cases had a 'genuine' injury with the rest labelled as 'emotional' cases that were treated rapidly and then sent straight back to the front line. The process was known as 'PIE' meaning proximity, immediacy and expectancy; treat the men close to the front line quickly and leave them under no illusion that they were expected to go back to the front line very soon. This was an attempt to undermine shell shock as a valid condition however, after the war, in 1921 the major combatants from all sides met to discuss shell shock. To their surprise they found that the experience was the same on all sides, people described re-experiencing the traumatic events via nightmares or flashbacks, they were often irritable, had difficulty concentrating or sleeping, they were hypervigilant and they tried, at all costs, to avoid situations that reminded them of the traumatic event or put them at risk of experiencing a similar trauma (ibid.).

Despite the consensus reached in 1921 the British government formed a committee of inquiry into shell shock that reported in 1922. Among its findings was that a loss of nervous mental control was not an opt-out from fighting and that soldiers experiencing such a condition would be treated separately from the ordinary wounded with an expectation that there would be a swift return to action (ibid.). It was obvious that the British Army wanted to send a clear message to soldiers that shell shock was not a condition that would lead to the sufferer being excused from fighting for any length of time. During the Second World War the British Army maintained their hard line on the emotional suffering of their soldiers but, wishing to move away from the concept of shell shock, now described soldiers who were traumatised as 'lacking moral fibre', 'LMF' for short. The American army used terms such as 'battle fatigue' or 'combat stress reaction' (CSR).

The psychiatric community reacted to this growing debate about emotional reactions to traumatic events when the American Psychiatric Association (APA) included the diagnosis of gross stress reaction in the first DSM, DSM-I, in 1952. This was however a very narrow definition of what conditions could cause trauma. The stress reaction had to be to traumatic events, such as disasters and combat, but the concept was limited by the fact that the sufferers were expected to make a full recovery within six months. If they still had symptoms after six months they were assigned a different diagnosis. The condition did not appear in the Second Edition of the DSM in 1968. As previously described, the concept of PTSD appears in the Third Edition of the DSM in 1980. In the intervening years a confluence of forces had influenced mainstream psychiatry including Holocaust survivors, returning veterans from the Vietnam War and associated anti-war activists and the women's movement highlighting sexual violence and trauma to women. These forces made it impossible for the condition to be ignored any longer.

The war poets and Craiglockhart hospital

It is unsurprising given the horrific nature of the conditions and the extent of the slaughter that took place during World War I that it inspired some incredibly visceral poetry from serving soldiers. This group of poets became known as the 'War poets' and it included Robert Graves, Siegfried Sassoon and Wilfred Owen. Sassoon and

Graves were fellow officers in the Royal Welch Fusiliers and Sassoon met Owen in 1917 at Craiglockhart hospital in Edinburgh where they were sent to receive treatment for 'shell shock'. Owen wrote a poem based heavily on his experiences at Craiglockhart entitled *Mental Cases* which opens with the lines:

Who are these? Why sit they here in twilight?
Wherefore rock they, purgatorial shadows,
Drooping tongues from jaws that slob their relish,
Baring teeth that leer like skulls' tongues wicked?

Owen's war experiences influenced him greatly. Initially he was contemptuous of the soldiers in his company describing them as knaves and expressionless lumps (Hibberd, 2003), however, his view of them changed when he experienced the reality of war. Four months into his time at the front, Owen became trapped under enemy fire for several days in a shell hole alone apart from the remains of another soldier. It was soon after this that he was evacuated from France and sent to Craiglockhart. While in hospital, as well as befriending his fellow poet Sassoon, who Owen admired greatly, he was also encouraged by his doctor, Arthur Brock, to translate his experiences into his poetry. Sassoon also made numerous comments and suggestions to Owen and it seems that the powerful anti-war poetry he became famous for was as a consequence of his experiences and the encouragement to write about them that he received at Craiglockhart (ibid.). Owen returned to France in July 1918 and was killed in action on the 4 November, exactly 1 week before the Armistice was signed.

Sassoon was deeply affected by the horrors he experienced in France and he appears to have become so affected that he engaged in numerous military actions during which he acted recklessly. His actions seemed almost suicidal in nature and because of this his men nicknamed him 'mad Jack' (Roberts, 2000). Back in England in 1917, on a period of convalescent leave, Sassoon refused to go back to France and instead issued an anti-war proclamation entitled *Finished with the War: A Soldier's Declaration*. In it he criticised the political errors and insincerities that had led to so much suffering for the troops and stated his intention to perform no further military duties (ibid.). It was Robert Graves, his friend and fellow poet, who convinced the government that Sassoon was suffering from 'shell shock' and it was agreed that he be sent to Craiglockhart rather than face a court martial (ibid.).

Sassoon nicknamed Craiglockhart 'Dottyville'; it was only open for 28 months from October 1916 to March 1919 and only treated officers, the other ranks were treated at other hospitals, such as Maghull which was built in 1911–1912 as the Moss Side State Institution and was originally built to house people with epilepsy. Though set up by the war office to treat shell shock, given their scepticism over the actual existence of the condition, there was considerable antagonism between the War Office and the doctors that ran them. When Owen and Sassoon were at Craiglockhart it was run by Major Bryce and the treatment regime was devised by Arthur John Brock, an Edinburgh clinician and medical historian. He devised an enlightened regime that he called 'ergotherapy' or 'cure by functioning'. He encouraged the patients to engage in numerous sporting and social activities. He also organised temporary teaching posts for them in local schools, jobs on local farms and also encouraged them to contribute to *The Hydra*, the hospital's in-house magazine. This gave them an opportunity to express and share their experiences and Owen became its editor for most of his time there and had his first published poems within its pages (Webb, 2006). The patients, Sassoon and Owen included, also received therapy from Brock, WHR Rivers, (made famous by his association with Sassoon as documented in Pat Barker's books especially the one entitled *Regeneration*) and other doctors. This was a humane approach to the traumatised and it encouraged them to discuss their repressed traumatic memories and was influenced by the psychoanalytical ideas of Sigmund Freud. His enlightened approach to treating shell shock cases was rare in other parts of Britain; doctors such as Lewis Yealland, who worked in London, did not believe it to be a real illness and he devised his treatment based on punishment, using electric shock treatment in severe cases.

The enlightened regime at Craiglockhart ended in November 1917 when the War Office removed Bryce and replaced him with Colonel Balfour Graham, a strict disciplinarian who altered the regime ensuring that the men had to do what they didn't like and were prevented from doing things that they did like. For example, those that disliked noise (common for traumatised soldiers who had been under fire) were given rooms on the main road and those who had been teachers or were poets were forbidden to use the library! Despite the fact that they were there due to their traumatic wartime experiences, in some senses, both Sassoon and Owen were lucky to be at Craiglockhart at the time they were as it was a much more enlightened therapeutic regime. Though Owen died in action, Sassoon was luckier. He returned to active service in 1918 until he was mistaken for a German soldier and shot in the head by a fellow British soldier, however, he survived and spent the rest of the war back in England.

Trauma and war

Another soldier of the First World War who was traumatised due to his experiences was the director, playwright and actor Arnold Ridley. Ironically, he became best known for his portrayal of Godfrey, the conscientious objector and bumbling elderly member of Walmington-on-Sea's Home Guard in *Dad's Army*. In real life he served in both world wars. In World War I he received shrapnel wounds in early 1916. By July he was back at the front in time for the Battle of the Somme. On the second occasion he went over the top, a lot of his battalion were cut down by machine gun fire. Ridley and other survivors found themselves in a German trench in which they had to fight their way along, using bayonets and grenades. During the fighting he had to deflect a German bayonet from his stomach into his groin, he then had a bayonet thrust through his left hand cutting his tendons and causing him to lose the use of three fingers – it took 15 operations to save his hand. He was also hit on the head with a rifle butt and for two years didn't realise it had fractured his skull. He experienced headaches for the rest of his life. He was discharged from the army in 1917 and suffered nightmares as a consequence of his experiences and, when acting on stage after the war, he was worried he would black out.

Despite these traumas, in 1923 he wrote the successful play *The Ghost Train*, and wrote other plays and acted between the wars. In 1939 he volunteered to rejoin the army at the outbreak of World

War II, however he stated that within hours of landing in France at Cherbourg he felt he was suffering from shell shock again and described it as like an 'inverted nightmare'. As is common for people who have PTSD, being back in the place where the trauma happened, or in a place that strongly reminds one of the trauma, provokes strong flashbacks and acute distress. Ridley, a modest man who did not speak often about his First World War experiences, was even more reticent about talking about his experiences in World War II as he so strongly associated them with re-experiencing emotional trauma. Despite enduring lifelong physical and emotional pain he was by all accounts a kind, gentle and decent man.

JD Salinger (1919–2010) was an American writer most famous for writing the novel *The Catcher in the Rye*. He also fought in World War II and saw action in France from April 1944 at D-Day onwards, including fighting at the Battle of the Bulge (Slawenski, 2012). Due to his linguistic skills he was assigned to a counter-intelligence division to interrogate German prisoners of war. As well as seeing active service, he and his regiment were in Aalen and Ellwangen, an area that contained a sub-camp of the Dachau concentration camp (it is thought that Salinger entered the camp, helping with the liberation of its victims). He never spoke directly about his wartime experiences, but it is documented that he spent time near the end of the war in an army hospital with combat stress which is what the American Army were then describing PTSD.

Salinger later used his wartime experiences in some of his short stories (ibid.). In one, *For Esme – with Love and Squalor*, one of the main characters is a traumatised American soldier and in another *A Perfect Day for Bananafish*, Seymour is a combat veteran who has been recently discharged from an army hospital and is causing concern to his wife by acting bizarrely and in an antisocial manner. Salinger is portraying how traumatised soldiers do not feel they can relate to civilian life or people around them, in the end Seymour takes his own life. It is not known if Salinger himself ever received any treatment other than his brief stay in an army hospital in Germany for the trauma he experienced in World War II.

It is often the case that people exposed to a traumatic event exhibit symptoms of trauma such as persistent remembering, avoidance or low mood soon after the trauma. However, sometimes people do not become symptomatic until years later. One such example is the British mountaineer Joe Simpson. Simpson and his climbing partner Simon Yates had climbed Siula Grande in the Peruvian Andes in 1985, but disaster struck as they descended from the summit. Simpson fell from an ice wall on the east face and smashed his right knee. They were still above 19,000 feet on the mountain and Yates tried to lower Simpson down one rope length at a time. After Yates had lowered him nearly 3,000 feet, Simpson slid off another edge and, and after holding the rope with frozen hands for nearly an hour, Yates couldn't take his weight any longer and was being pulled off the mountain. He had to decide whether to be pulled off and fall with Simpson or cut the rope, leaving Simpson to fall but saving himself. He chose to cut the rope. Miraculously Simpson fell into a crevasse and landed on a ledge. He was able to crawl up a snow cone out of the crevasse and he then crawled for three days in a semi-delirious state back to his camp. Simpson wrote a fascinating book about the incident called *Touching the Void*. He needed six operations on his knee before he could climb again. However, he did not experience PTSD until years later in 2002. This happened when he returned to Peru to make a film based on the book and, being there, brought all the memories flooding back. He has subsequently said that it felt like the 'accident had happened only five minutes ago'.

In 1993 the tennis star, Monica Seles, was stabbed at a tournament in Hamburg by a disturbed tennis fan who wanted the German tennis player, Steffi Graff, back as world number one. The assailant used a nine-inch serrated-edged boning knife. He only managed to plunge it in one and a half inches before he was tackled by people close by. Seles was only 19 years of age at the time and, though the physical injury healed quickly, the mental ones took a lot longer. It was 27 months before she returned to action. She has talked openly in the media about how traumatised this attack left her and how she feared returning to play tennis suffering from nightmares and flashbacks. She received therapy from her sports psychologist Dr Jerry May; he encouraged her to set small goals, initially asking her to just walk around her own garden. He also taught her relaxation techniques to help her control the distressing emotions that accompanied the nightmares she was experiencing. She gradually recovered enough to return to top class tennis.

Unfortunately, there are many people who have been trauma-tised by wars, famine and political instability in many regions of the world. Many of these people try to escape the source of their trauma in their home country and seek a better life elsewhere. However, in the process of travelling, many experience further traumas and, when they do arrive at what they hope is a safe haven, they are often subject to yet more trauma including uncertainty over their status, discrimination, detention, dispersal, destitution and denial of the right to work (McColl et al., 2008). However, the World Health Organization (WHO, 2013) in its guidelines on conditions specifically related to stress, pointed out that those guidelines that do exist have been developed for high-income country health systems, are for use in specialised care and are not based on a systematic review of the evidence. Therefore, they developed their guidelines (ibid.) to help people who are working in non-specialist (not mental health) services that are likely to have first contact with people who have experienced a traumatic event.

Treatments for PTSD

The most recent National Institute for Health and Care Excellence (NICE, 2018) pathway for PTSD in the UK begins by advising ser-vices to screen people at risk of developing PTSD after a major disaster. It also advises that services screen refugees and asylum seekers who present to mental health services. The guidelines advise watchful waiting for people who have mild symptoms and have had them for less than four weeks. However, it is often the case, espe-cially for people who have travelled long distances, that they do not come into contact with services until many weeks after experienc-ing trauma. It is often the case that by the time refugees and asylum seekers reach services, PTSD has become well established and, in periods of acute distress, people can be very harmful to themselves. In such circumstances a whole team approach – whereby the person is under a service such as a community mental health team – is best able to manage the risks and meet their needs which may include housing, benefits, social isolation as well as the trauma focussed therapy they need.

A review (Slobodin & de Jong, 2015) of studies into the effectiveness of interventions designed especially for traumatised asylum seekers and refugees found that, despite the shortage of frameworks available to clinicians attempting to tailor interventions to these groups, interventions such as culturally sensitive CBT and Narrative Exposure Therapy (NET), which combines CBT with testimony therapy, have been effective with refugees.

The NICE (2018) guidelines for PTSD recommend one of two treatments for people who have had persistent symptoms for more than three months. They are: trauma-focussed CBT, and Eye Movement Desensitisation and Reprocessing (EMDR) – the WHO (2013) also recommends CBT but states that the quality of the evidence for EMDR being effective is very low. However, both CBT and EMDR have been proven to be effective for the treatment of trauma (Bisson et al., 2007). The main focus of EMDR is on the distressing memories that accompany a traumatic experience (Ter Heide et al., 2016). It has several phases of treatment with a focus on a three-pronged approach; past memories, present disturbance and future actions. The therapy aims to identify past memories that are associated with a traumatic event that have led to a current negative self-belief and associated negative emotion. For example, a person may have been involved in a natural disaster and a memory of it is associated with the belief 'I am in danger' but, in EMDR therapy, they will be asked to generate a new belief such as 'I am safe now'. In some respects it has similarities to CBT in that it identifies negative beliefs and tries to undermine the strength of them and replace them with a more balanced, evidenced view. The main difference is that during the desensitisation phase while dealing with the negative beliefs associated with a traumatic memory, the person is asked to engage in bilateral stimulation most commonly in the form of repeated eye movements (ibid.). Bilateral stimulation is a core element of EMDR and is stimuli, either visual, tactile or auditory, that occurs in a rhythmic side-to-side pattern.

Though EMDR has been proven to be effective this is not without controversy, as some (Salkovskis, 2002) have argued that what is effective about EMDR is those elements it shares in common with CBT and that the eye movements are irrelevant. However, the World Health Organization (WHO, 2013) identified clear distinctions between the two approaches noting that EMDR is based on the idea that negative thoughts and emotions are the result of unprocessed memories and that, unlike trauma focussed CBT, it does not involve detailed descriptions of the event, direct challenging of beliefs or direct exposure. The WHO (ibid.) after reviewing the data found moderate evidence to support the beneficial effect in decreasing symptom severity for both individual trauma focussed CBT and group trauma focused CBT. Further, they also found that in certain cultural situations EMDR has been interpreted as witchcraft, increasing stress and anxiety for some of its recipients.

When it comes to the evidence base for medication to treat PTSD, the WHO (ibid.) conducted a review of the literature and could find no studies of randomised controlled trials (RCTs) of pharmacotherapy for adults with acute traumatic stress ('acute' meaning stress occurring within the first month of experiencing trauma). They therefore recommended that antidepressants and benzodiazepines should not be offered to adults to reduce acute traumatic stress symptoms in the first month after a potentially traumatic event. They similarly found no evidence for the use of pharmacotherapy for children and adolescents with acute traumatic stress.

The WHO (ibid.) explored the evidence base for the use of pharmacotherapy for adults with established PTSD and found a small, but statistically significant, beneficial effect in adults. As the effect size was small, the WHO recommended that antidepressants should not be offered as a first-line treatment and should only be offered if CBT with a trauma focus, EMDR and stress management have failed or are not available; or if the person also has a co-morbid moderate-to-severe depressive illness. They looked specifically at antidepressants that were most likely available now or in the next five years in non-specialised health care in low- and middle-income countries. This was done to ensure that the review analysed the data of what is available on a worldwide basis. Antidepressants that are still on license are a lot more expensive than those that are off license and termed 'generic' and as such are beyond the means of many parts of the world.

As has been stated in this chapter, the symptoms of anxiety are a normal response to, and help us deal with, challenging situations. It is only when our response is disproportionate to the actual situation that people develop problems functioning on a day-to-day basis.

As this chapter has shown, anxiety disorders are very common, they are also very treatable. A combination of a talking therapy, healthy lifestyle choices such as a good diet, exercise and moderate alcohol consumption and, in some cases, the use of various classes of anti-depressants, can have a significant positive impact on the degree of anxiety that an individual experiences and help them on their journey to recovery.

2

Depression

Dejection

> A grief without a pang, void, dark and drear,
> A stifled, drowsy, unimpassioned grief,
> Which finds no natural outlet, no relief
> In word, or sigh, or tear (Coleridge, 1802)

Depression is one of the most common mental disorders in the world. It is a leading cause of disability worldwide, and is a major contributor to the overall global burden of disease. Globally, more than 300 million people of all ages suffer from depression and more women are affected than men. It used to be thought that depression was rare in Africa but cross-cultural views have changed in the past 60 years and it is now accepted that rates in parts of Africa are actually higher than in Western societies (Kleinman & Cohen, 2001). Many studies have demonstrated that rates of depression correlate strongly with poverty, illiteracy, trauma, conflict and gender. Such factors are unfortunately very prevalent across many parts of the world.

The stigma attached to mental health issues has meant that rates of depression in some parts of the world were surprisingly low (even in societies with high rates of suicide, which seemed puzzling) but this has begun to shift in recent years. In Japan, for example, people did not look upon depression favourably because the Japanese term for depression *'utsubyou'* was hardly known outside of clinical circles and had a restricted meaning of severe depression (Ihara, 2012). In an attempt to lessen the stigma attached to depression (and increase sales of newer-generation antidepressants) pharmaceutical companies coined the term 'kokoro no kaze' the literal meaning of which is 'cold of the soul'. This was in order to associate depression closer to everyday illnesses, such as the common cold, rather than a severe mental illness and, consequently, sales of antidepressants increased sixfold between 1998 and 2006 (ibid.). However, as has been pointed out (ibid.) this is misleading as people would expect to take a cold remedy for only a few days but may take medication for depression for at least several months, and possibly even years.

The main features of depression are persistent sadness, a loss of interest in activities that are usually enjoyable, reduced energy level, and an inability to carry out daily activities. However, in some parts of the developing world somatic complaints (medically unexplained physical symptoms) such as headaches and neck pain are more commonly described than emotional symptoms (WHO, 2017a). For a diagnosis of depression to be considered the person has to feel this way for at least two weeks. Other common symptoms include: a change in appetite; sleeping more, or less; anxiety; reduced concentration; restlessness; feelings of worthlessness, guilt, or hopelessness; and thoughts of self-harm or suicide. Approximately 800,000 people worlwide die due to suicide every year and suicide is the second leading cause of death in 15–29-year-olds (ibid.). Depression is a condition of varying severity but is closely related to suicide. Many people who experience a mild, depressive episode recover without seeking treatment and many of those who experience a moderate episode recover with the help of antidepressants and possibly a talking therapy and do not generally need to see trained mental health professionals (in those parts of the world where such professionals are available).

Depression results from a complex interaction of social, psychological and biological factors. There are interrelationships between depression and physical health. For example, cardiovascular disease can lead to depression and vice versa. People who have gone through adverse life events (e.g. unemployment, bereavement, psychological trauma) are more likely to develop depression. Depression can, in turn, lead to more stress and dysfunction and worsen the affected person's life situation and the depression itself. In 2017 the World Health Organization's (ibid.) fact sheet on depression identified that despite the existence of known, effective treatments for depression, fewer than half of those affected in the world (in many countries, fewer than ten per cent) received such treatments. Barriers to effective care included a lack of resources, lack of trained healthcare providers and the social stigma associated with mental disorders. Another barrier identified was that people who are depressed are often not correctly diagnosed and that this occurred in countries of all income levels. Interestingly, they also found the converse to be true, that people who weren't depressed were often misdiagnosed and prescribed antidepressants.

From the earliest times when humans described their emotional states in antiquity considerable elements of what we would recognise as depression today came under the broader heading of *melancholia*. Melancholia, as has been described in the Introduction, was thought to exist due an excess of black bile. The Romans thought that melancholy could lead to the more serious condition of *mania* (Pietikainen, 2015). Though descriptions of melancholia do not correspond exactly to our modern concept of depression, they include within them descriptions of sadness that would be recognisable to us as very similar to the depression we understand today. The publication in the seventeenth century of Robert Burton's *The Anatomy of Melancholy* (1621) helped make it a fashionable disease in this period and his description of the melancholic person as one who is 'dull, sad and ill-disposed' is one we would recognise as true of people with depression today (Scull, 2015). Burton also demonstrated a key insight when he said in his book 'I write of melancholy by being busy to avoid melancholy' as encouraging people to keep a routine of activity is often part of a treatment package when working with people with depression to this day (see Figure 2.1).

'Depression' is a relatively recent addition to the English language dating back to the eighteenth century (Rousseau, 2000) and was apparently first coined by Samuel Johnson. Rousseau (ibid.) describes the older term 'melancholia' as a pre-medicalised category associated with humoral theory and religious theories of satanic possession and therefore distinct from the modern medicalised concept of depression. However, he also noted that the older version did contain enough characteristics central to the newer one to be able to conceptualise a continuous history of depression despite their clear

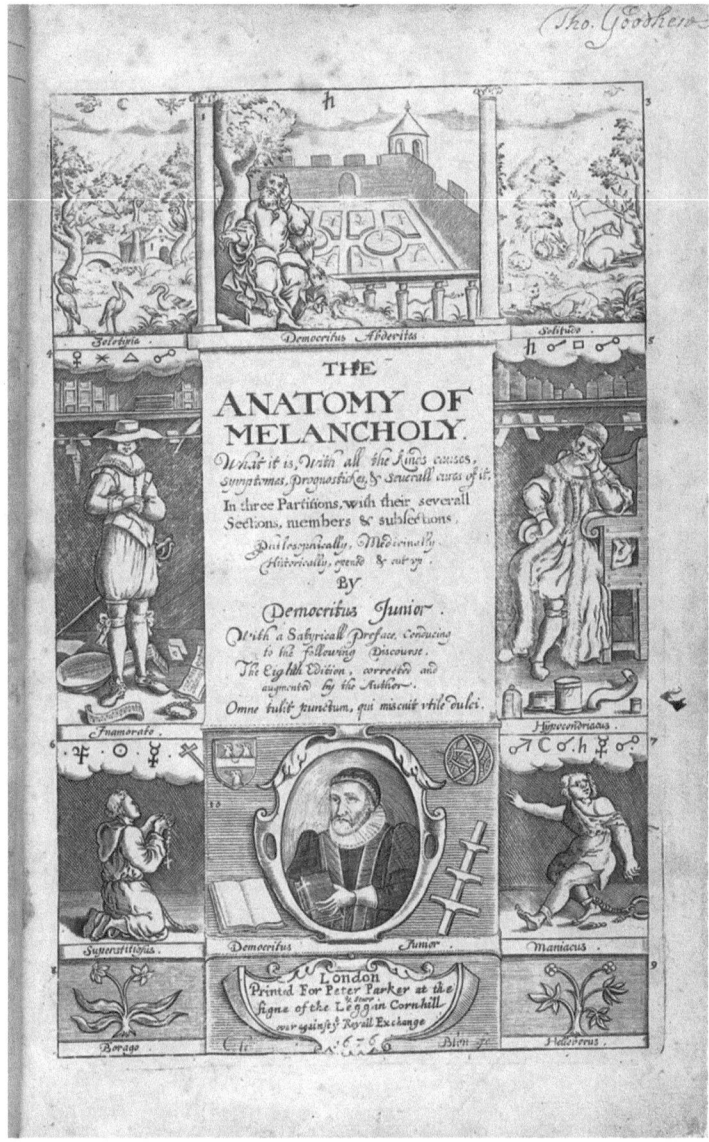

Figure 2.1 Robert Burton: *The anatomy of melancholy*; London: Peter Parker, 1676. Frontispiece engraved by C. le Blon. (Wellcome Collection).

differences. He also argued that such an approach would narrow the history of depression as it entails ignoring the significant differences between melancholy and depression. However, that melancholia as a pre-medicalised concept and our medicalised concepts of mental illnesses have a significant degree of crossover throughout history is clear, especially in the case of depression. This is because the main focus of it as an illness lies in human emotions and, despite the different historical and cultural contexts that shape the ways in which we express our emotions, what we actually *feel* is unchanged through time.

An example of an individual who saw melancholia not as satanic possession but as an illness is Johann Weyer (or Wier 1515–1588). The Dutch physician and demonologist opposed the burning of women as witches claiming they were not worshippers of the devil but were sufferers of melancholia or some other form of madness. By challenging the religious views then dominant he fanned the early flames of rationality. Weyer was, for a time, the private physician to the Duke of Cleves (brother of Anne of Cleves who was, for six months, the fourth wife of King Henry VIII) who himself suffered from depression. The treatments that Weyer would have used at that time were the usual array of bleeding, cupping, emetics and laxatives designed to restore balance between the four humours.

Oliver Cromwell, one of the leading figures in the English Civil War that led to the execution of King Charles I of England, was born in 1599 into a wealthy family and is known to have experienced a considerable episode of depression. Unfortunately for Cromwell, his uncle, Sir Oliver, had dissipated much of the family fortune and this was compounded by the fact that his father, Robert, was a younger son and so inherited little – meaning that his particular branch of the Cromwell family were, by all accounts, the poor relations. He was, however, well connected and when he was first elected to the House of Commons in 1628 he found (Hill, 1988) nine of his cousins there! Unfortunately he became embroiled in a dispute about the control of the corporation of his seat at Huntingdon and was accused of making disgraceful speeches and was hauled in front of the Privy Council where the judgement went against him. Having experienced a political defeat, he sold nearly all his property in Huntingdon and moved elsewhere in the county where he lived in reduced circumstances as a farmer. Around this time he sought treatment from the famed physician Sir Theodore Mayerne for various physical and emotional ailments and it is recorded that he was treated for melancholia (ibid.). Mayerne was an alchemist and is known to have used a vast array of chemical compounds in his treatments. It's possible that the stress of becoming an MP, the later political disputes and his economic misfortunes led to Cromwell's mood lowering, though there are few surviving letters from this period. What *is* known is that this was also the period of his conversion to a radical form of Protestantism known as *Puritanism* from which he gained great emotional and spiritual comfort. His return to a position of higher social status only occurred in the mid-1630s via a family inheritance (see Figure 2.2).

Almost 200 years after Cromwell, the political philosopher John Stuart Mill (1806–1873) wrote his autobiography in which he

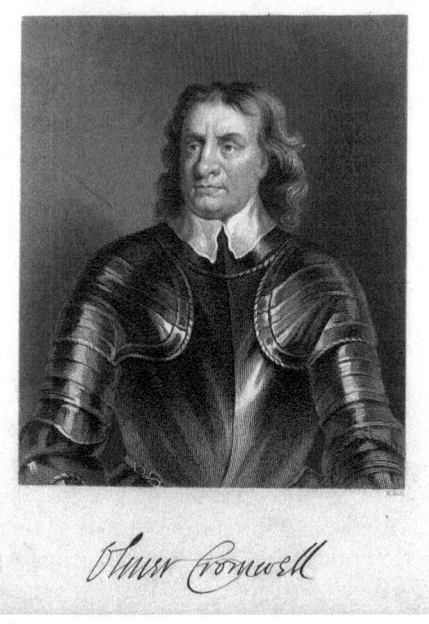

Figure 2.2 Portrait of Oliver Cromwell, with facsimile signature by W. Holl. (Wellcome Collection).

described an episode of depression in 1826 where he experienced no pleasure or enjoyment in life. He described the situation as like a cloud that grew thicker as the months progressed. His account of his crisis in his mental history, as he himself put it, would be familiar to anyone experiencing a depressive episode, he describes gaining no enjoyment from pastimes such as reading and music, both of which he usually enjoyed greatly. He further describes his distress as neither interesting nor respectable, indicating a sensitivity to the stigma associated with mental health problems, and so he did not speak to other people about it (Oyebode, 2010). His account of his recovery is also interesting, he describes reading a memoire in which he read of the death of the author's father and how this affected the whole family. Mill states that he was moved to tears and that this expression of emotion demonstrated to him that he wasn't devoid of emotion as he had begun to think. He then describes gradually gaining a degree of enjoyment in day-to-day experiences and activities and that the cloud which had been over him, gradually disappeared.

Many politicians have suffered from depression and Davidson et al. (2006) note that there seems to be a particularly high rate among American presidents. Their analysis of secondary sources found depression to be present in a number of them including Abraham Lincoln, Woodrow Wilson, Calvin Coolidge and John Quincey Adams. The same has been found to be the case for a significant number of British Prime Ministers including Benjamin Disraeli, David Lloyd George, Neville Chamberlain and Winston Churchill (Davidson, 2011). Much has been written about Churchill's (1874–1965) own description of his depressive episodes as his 'black dog' (which is an ancient metaphor for depression and melancholy with a history stretching back to the Romans) and Churchill himself wrote about how he took up painting at a time in his life when he was experiencing depression and anxiety and found it very therapeutic – though, as his episodes of depression reoccurred, it obviously wasn't sufficient to keep depression at bay.

David Lloyd George (1863–1945), a contemporary of Churchill, became prime minister in 1916 in the middle of the First World War. Like Churchill, he was a successful wartime prime minister but also a deeply complicated figure with a complex personality. He had been a successful reforming minister being a leading figure in the introduction of the National Insurance Act in 1911 that laid the foundations of the welfare state in Britain. His government passed many socially progressive reforms near the end of and after World War I not least among them an Education Act (1918) that raised the school leaving age to 14 and The Representation of the People Act (1918) that extended the right to vote franchise to all adult males (over the age of 21) and most women (over the age of 30). It was also documented that he experienced several episodes of depression in his life. These were usually as a consequence of stressful life events, for example, he suffered a severe grief reaction in 1907 after the death of his daughter, Mair, during an appendectomy; from which, by all accounts, he never fully recovered. A depressive episode occurred in 1913 after he was caught up in a financial scandal when he bought shares whilst privy to inside information on future contracts the company would be awarded (ibid.). The ensuing enquiry took a great emotional toll on him that lasted for several months. He suffered a further episode near the end of his premiership around 1921–1922 when he was much less influential politically in the, then, coalition government. There were a number of other factors to this including: the worsening economic situation in Britain; the War of Independence in Ireland (1919–1921); and the growing financial scandal that gathered around him when he was found to be selling honours and titles for personal gain. There were other obvious periods when he was under great stress, especially during the war due to the massive loss of life at the front, though there is no evidence (ibid.) that he experienced a depressive episode during the war. What was noticeable at times of stress was that Lloyd George experienced a number of physical ailments when he was stressed or depressed (ibid.). As was mentioned earlier, experiencing physical pain for which no physical cause can be found when low in mood is quite common in some cultures and what Lloyd George's case demonstrates is that such presentations are also found in Western populations. In his case these ailments included at various times muscle weakness, muscle pain and nervous exhaustion which tended to resolve after he had a period of rest and/or his stress levels reduced.

Other groups that seem very prone to depression are sportsmen/women and writers. One group of sports people with a particularly high rate of suicide is cricketers and, in a fascinating book on the subject, David Frith (2001) speculates on the reasons why this is so, some of which would be the same for any person (e.g. financial insecurity, relationship breakdown). He further adds the fact that many cricketers seem unable to cope when their careers have ended and they no longer have the camaraderie of the team, the excitement of playing or the recognition and rewards that accompany the game. These factors also hold true for other sports, such as football, where there have also been a number of cases of depression though footballers seem more willing now to talk about their insecurities and mental health problems than previous generations did.

Frith (ibid.) identified over 150 cricketers who committed suicide in little over a century and countless others who had experienced significant depressive episodes including among them Phil Tuffnell, Graham Dilley, Jack Russell, Marcus Trescothick and Jonathon Trott. An interesting cultural aside that Frith (ibid.) describes is that, while the rate of suicide in Asia among cricketers is negligible, the same cannot be said for cricket *fans* and he recounts a number of cases where cricket fans in India, Pakistan and Sri Lanka have committed suicide after their team have had a bad result.

There have been a considerable number of writers including, Charles Dickens, Leo Tolstoy, Charlotte Perkins Gilman, George Elliot, Herman Hesse, Jack Kerouac, Hans Fallada, F. Scott Fitzgerald, Tennessee Williams, Virginia Wolfe and Sylvia Plath who have experienced depressive episodes. Both Wolfe and Plath committed suicide whilst in a state of depression. Perkins Gilman also committed suicide though hers was a decision made due to her having terminal cancer rather than due to an episode of depression. Our view on which occupations are closely associated with depression could be skewed, however, by the fact that people in occupations in the public eye, such as politicians and writers, are going to be noticed. The Health and Safety Executive figures for work-related stress, depression and anxiety in Great Britain for 2018 show that 526,000 people identified themselves as having work-related mental health problems and the occupations with the highest rates were those working in human health and social work activities (HSE, 2018).

That adversity can have a shattering effect on a person's emotional state and provoke a depressive episode is clear and a good example is the ten day disappearance of the writer Agatha Christie in

1926. She became depressed due to a combination of the recent loss of her mother, overwork and her husband's announcement that he wanted a divorce as he was having an affair. An extensive manhunt took place over the ensuing ten days until she was found in a hotel in Harrogate registered under the name of her husband's lover. Christie made no mention of this episode in her later autobiography.

A more tragic case is that of the black actor, singer and civil rights campaigner Paul Robeson. Robeson appeared in movies and on Broadway, he also marched in hunger marches with Welsh miners, went to Spain during the Spanish Civil war and was outspoken against racism. Indeed in the mid-1930s he appeared in the West End in London in *Toussaint Louverture* a play about the eighteenth century black revolutionary leader of the slave revolt in Haiti, written by the black Marxist C.L.R James. This was the first time a play was performed in Britain where black actors performed in a play written by a black playwright (Hogsberg, 2010). He also became sympathetic to communism and visited the Soviet Union a number of times. After the Second World War and the rise of McCarthyism in the USA Robeson was blacklisted for his political views and he was denied a passport and banned from leaving the USA, cutting off both his sources of income in America and abroad. Unable to work in America or abroad he also could not attend any political events around the world, curtailing both his ability to earn money and to be a political activist. His recordings and films were also removed from public distribution. In 1956 he was called to appear in front of the House Un-American Activities Committee (HUAC) and after he and his wife refused to sign an affidavit denying they were communists his passport was revoked and, though having never been charged with any offence, found a number of his civil rights denied to him.

Robeson was given back his passport in 1958 after campaigns by others in a similar position and by organisations committed to fighting McCarthyism. This meant he could once again travel the world performing and in 1959 he appeared in England in *Othello* for the Royal Shakespeare Company. Unfortunately by 1961 he began to experience significant depressive symptoms brought on by the years of stress of being blacklisted, persecuted, closely monitored by the CIA and FBI and slandered by various US government agencies (Goodman, 2013). He also experienced paranoid ideas which, given the degree of surveillance and persecution he had experienced, is not surprising. He suffered depressive episodes whilst in Moscow and London and, during one of these in London, he became suicidal and was admitted to the Priory hospital. Here he was given high doses of tranquilising drugs and during a two year stay received 54 doses of electroconvulsive therapy (ECT). His health broken, he returned to the USA in 1963. Tragically, now in poor health he was unable to take any meaningful part in the civil rights movement that grew in the US throughout the 1960s, instead he lived quietly out of the public eye until his death in 1976.

Electroconvulsive therapy, unlike the other early 'shock' treatments such as insulin coma therapy, is still in use today. Initially developed in the 1930s it was then used for a range of conditions including depression, schizophrenia and bipolar disorder. A convulsive therapy was first considered as a treatment for psychosis based on the incorrect observation by the Hungarian neuropathologist Ladislas von Meduna that schizophrenia and epilepsy did not occur together (Shorter, 1997). Initially it wasn't electricity that was used to induce a seizure – Meduna used camphor dissolved in oil. He had a positive response in several of his subjects but these were a particular subgroup of schizophrenic patients, people in a catatonic state. This means they were in a state of motor immobility and stupor and, luckily for Meduna, this is a condition that is actually very responsive to induced seizures. Camphor was inconsistent in producing fits so he experimented with the drug Mertrazol which was more reliable but unfortunately, as well as producing a considerable degree of anxiety in his subjects, it also produced side effects including vomiting, joint dislocations, heart damage and even the occasional death (Scull, 2015).

The search for a safer way to induce seizures was completed in 1938 by two Italian psychiatrists who were experimenting by passing an electrical current through dogs. One of them, Lucio Bini, discovered that the safest way was by passing the current through the dog's temples (Shorter, 1997). They subsequently experimented on humans and found that the effect (a convulsion) was easier and cheaper to induce with an electrical current than the drugs that were then in use. Bini and his colleague, Ugo Cerletti, tried it three times at increasing voltage on their first patient until they induced a tonic-clonic seizure. Apparently after 11 applications of ECT the patient, psychotic on admission, was well enough to go home though apparently some of his symptoms returned several months later (ibid.). Like other supposed 'cures' before it the exaggerated claims of its effectiveness ensured that ECT quickly became popular across Europe and the USA. One of the first problems that the early pioneers noticed was the violent convulsions sometimes resulted in bone fractures for the patient and so 'modified ECT', where a muscle relaxant was also used to prevent the fractures, was introduced from 1942 (Scull, 2015).

ECT is still used today, though far more sparingly than in the decades before the 1970s. Though it has been in use continuously since 1938 how it works is still unclear – it is thought that it may stimulate the release of some of the chemicals in the brain associated with lifting low mood, it is also thought that it may help the growth of new cells and nerve pathways within the brain (RCP, 2015). Of all the treatments currently in use for mental health issues, ECT is probably the most contentious. There are a number of reasons for this. Though ECT does lift mood it can also produce short-term side effects such as headaches and longer-term side effects such as problems with one's memory. The writer Ernest Hemmingway had several courses of ECT in 1960 and 1961 but, two days after on his release in June 1960, he committed suicide by shooting himself in the head. Scull (2015) suggests that this was in part due to the damaging effect of ECT on Hemmingway's memory and hence his ability to write. However, it is also true that Hemmingway's talent had been damaged by years of excessive alcohol abuse and that his father had also committed suicide by shooting himself and, at a later date, so did his brother, Leicester. His sister, Ursula, also committed suicide as did a granddaughter, Margaux. Therefore, there is a strong familial link to severe mental health problems and suicide that cannot be attributed solely to ECT. Another point of view is that, as is often seen in clinical practice, after several sessions of ECT people regain a degree of volition they had lost when severely depressed. Unfortunately, they are still often very low in mood and continue to have suicidal thoughts; making this a risky period in the recovery process.

The rise of a radical critique of psychiatric practices in the 1960s the antipsychiatry movement did lead to increased attacks on ECT and this first was given impetus by the publication of the book *One Flew Over The Cuckoo's Nest* written by Ken Kesey in 1962. The film version in 1975 especially portrayed ECT as a method of punishing and controlling the patients in a negative way. This film had a profoundly negative effect on the public's perception of mental healthcare in general but of ECT in particular. At the same time the advances in pharmacological treatments meant that many psychiatrists also hoped that medication could be used instead of the more rudimentary technique of passing an electrical current through the individual's brain. However, ECT is still available because it does work and, in cases of severe depression that are often resistant to antidepressant medication, ECT should still be considered since the risk of suicide or self-neglect from severe depression is significant.

Treatments for depression

Prevention programmes have been shown to be effective in reducing rates of depression. Effective community approaches to prevent depression include school-based programmes to enhance a pattern of positive thinking in children and adolescents. Interventions for parents of children with behavioural problems may reduce parental depressive symptoms and improve outcomes for their children. Exercise programmes for the elderly can also be effective in depression prevention.

There are effective treatments for moderate and severe depression. The two main treatment approaches that are used are *antidepressant medication* and *talking therapies,* most clinicians agree that a combination of the two is the most effective approach to take. Psychological treatments include behavioural activation, cognitive behavioural therapy (CBT) and interpersonal psychotherapy (IPT). For some people with milder forms of depression, self-help books (bibliotherapy) or access to internet or computer administered varieties of therapy may be sufficient to treat their low mood. This is important as not all parts of the world have access to therapists so bibliotherapy may fill part of this deficit. Behaviour Therapy (BT) along with CBT and IPT have all proven to be effective in robust randomised controlled trials, this is because they all use measures of effectiveness such as the

Beck Depression Inventory (BDI) to measure the impact of treatment on the individual. At its simplest level, CBT helps people identify the negative automatic thoughts that people with low mood generate and then tries to help the individual generate more balanced thoughts (Williams, 1999). This is accompanied by challenging information processing biases such as mind-reading (I know people think I'm bad at my job), predicting the future (if I try x activity I know I will perform badly) and catastrophising (if I go to such an event it will be a disaster). People who are low in mood tend to have a more negative appraisal of themselves, other people and the world around them. CBT attempts to challenge these negative cognitions partly by questioning and partly by setting up behavioural experiments that test the individual's negative predictions.

As with the accidental finding that the antihistamine, Chlorpromazine, was effective as an antipsychotic the discovery of antidepressants was equally serendipitous. When testing a derivative of chlorpromazine, imipramine, as a potential antipsychotic in the late 1950s it was observed to not have any antipsychotic effect but it did elevate the mood of patients that were also depressed (Hillhouse & Porter, 2015). This observation led to the discovery of one of the first classes of antidepressants – due to its chemical structure imipramine and similar drugs became known as *tricyclic* antidepressants. It wasn't described in terms of its mode of action because at the time of the discovery of its effectiveness as an antidepressant its mode of action was unknown. At around the same time a drug used to treat tuberculosis, iproniazid, was also noted to have positive effects on the patient's mood. Over time is was discovered that it elevated mood by preventing the break down in the brain of the monoamines serotonin, dopamine, epinephrine and norepinephrine and, as such, it and other drugs working in the same mode of action became known as Mono Amine Oxidase Inhibiters (MAOIs). Both tricyclics and MAOIs are effective antidepressants that work in different ways to elevate the amount of amines, especially serotonin, in the brain. Unfortunately both are also highly toxic in overdose and, given the propensity of people to take impulsive or planned overdoses whilst depressed, this was a serious issue that was only solved by the later synthesis of a third group of antidepressants, the Selective Serotonin Reuptake Inhibitors (SSRIs). However, SSRIs can cause side effects such as agitation and restlessness that have made some depressed people become more desperate and there have been cases recorded of increased suicidality caused by this class of antidepressant too. Broadly speaking each class of antidepressant confers similar antidepressant effects though their mechanisms of action differ.

Despite the efficacy of antidepressants for some people, unfortunately they do not work for everyone. External factors such as adverse life events and trauma have been demonstrated to alter the structure and function of our brains. The fact that internal factors such as our own thoughts can also influence our brain chemistry and how we feel means that the causes and factors that maintain depression are multiple and complex. Despite this, antidepressants are big business – in the UK in 2014 over 57 million antidepressant prescription items were dispensed and in 2016 antidepressants saw the greatest numeric rise of all British National Formulary (BNF) therapeutic areas for prescription items dispensed in the community in England (NHS Digital, 2017).

Depression in women

Studies have shown that women are almost twice as likely to suffer from depression as men and 70 per cent of people who receive ECT are women (Kennedy et al., 2007). Twenty per cent of women experience some depression during pregnancy and postnatal mood disturbances are common. Postnatal depression is very common and many famous women have spoken about it and what helped them – for the actor Gwyneth Paltrow it was increased exercise, whereas when the actor Courtney Cox felt low after the birth of her daughter her doctor discovered that her hormone levels were low and she was prescribed progesterone which, alongside the support of friends and family, helped her recover. Brooke Shields the actor has spoken about how she felt no connection to her baby daughter and felt depressed and alienated from those around her. She has written a book *Down Came the Rain: My Journey Through Postpartum Depression* (Shields, 2005) in which she details her developing low mood and how a combination of family support, therapy and antidepressants helped her to recover.

Challenging the stigma of depression

As with almost all mental health issues, there is still a considerable degree of stigma attached to being depressed, it has historically been perceived by some as a sign of weakness. This is especially true in some cultures, for example, in Japan and China where it has been difficult to voice emotional problems and symptoms have usually been couched in terms of physical symptoms. Challenging the stigma associated with depression has been boosted by having people who would in general be thought of as successful stand up and say that they have experienced depression. Over the last few years a number of such individuals *have* spoken about their experiences. In 2015 during a debate in the House of Commons about mental health, the Labour MP Jeff Smith disclosed his own struggles with depression. Like Brooke Shields, the singer Sheryl Crow has spoken about how she tried a combination of antidepressants and therapy but then replaced the antidepressants with exercise to help her overcome depression. Alastair Campbell is a passionate campaigner for better funding for mental health services and a challenger of the stigma around mental health issues – he has described the stigma around it as the last great taboo. He is a British journalist, political commentator, author and former Downing Street press secretary under the Tony Blair premiership. He has used these skills to effectively describe his own experiences of alcoholism and depression, of how he had a depressive episode so severe he was also psychotic and needed hospitalising. He has spoken candidly about his experiences in numerous pieces in the press, on TV, in TED (technology, entertainment and design) talks and especially in a film entitled *Cracking Up*. All of these help to normalise the emotional breakdown of depression under the stress of life events. He has also spoken about how resilient people are and how, sometimes, what one learns from the worse experiences in life can increase a person's resilience and help them grow. By challenging stigma people such as Sheryl Crow and Alastair Campbell make it easier for other people to be open about how they feel which is the first step towards seeking the help they may need.

3

Dementia

The term 'dementia' has a long history. It originally had a broader definition and was thought of both medically and philosophically as describing a process of mental deterioration associated with old age (Earlstein, 2016). Many of the ancient Greek philosophers saw it as an inevitable process associated with ageing. The ancient Greek philosopher Pythagoras divided the human life span into six distinct phases and in the latter two he described them as the 'senium', a period of physical and mental decay. Up to the eighteenth century dementia continued to have a broad meaning of psychological incompetence regardless of age (Berrios, 2008). However, during the nineteenth century psychiatrists began to study the disease and its meaning began to narrow. Studies of the brains of people who had died of dementia by numerous psychiatrists in the latter part of the nineteenth century had identified a number of changes present in the brain including, atrophy of affected regions, plaques, tangles and arteriosclerotic changes.

The publication of a paper by the German psychiatrist, Alois Alzheimer, in 1907 in which he described these degenerative changes in a 51-year-old woman was at that time only remarkable because of the relatively young age of the patient. For example in the same year the Czech psychiatrist Oskar Fischer published a paper describing the conditions of 16 patients and provided the first description of the neuritic plaques found in dementia (Goedert, 2009). The difference was that Alzheimer worked with one of the most influential psychiatrists of the time, Emile Kraepelin, and in 1910 Kraepelin published the eighth edition of his text book on psychiatry in which, in his section on senile dementia, he described the condition as 'Alzheimer's disease', the reasons for this are unclear. Also, as Kraepelin had noted the young age of the Alzheimer's patient, for generations after that many held the false assumption that younger patients had Alzheimer's disease while older patients had dementia, when actually they were the same condition. It is now known that it is actually Frontotemporal Dementia (FTD) that often occurs at an earlier age. FTD covers a range of conditions but what occurs in all of them is damage to frontal and temporal lobes in the brain.

'Dementia' is not one illness but rather an umbrella term for a number of conditions and is therefore better described as a *syndrome*. It is a progressive condition that affects the higher cognitive functions of the brain including memory, thinking, language, learning capacity and orientation, among others. Also dementia is not, as some people think, a normal part of ageing, it occurs when the brain is affected by disease (Earlstein, 2016).

The causes of dementia remain unclear though it is thought to be multifactorial involving a complex interaction of genetic, life style and environmental factors. However; having said that, the most important component of dementia is that these diseases most often occur as people age. As people in large parts of the world now live much longer than they did in previous generations, prevalence rates for dementia have risen significantly in recent decades. In some parts of the world dementia is dealt with by physicians, not mental health clinicians, as it is thought of as a brain disease and not a mental disorder. However, dementia is more than a brain disease as it affects the whole person and, for that reason, it has often fallen under the auspices of mental health services. It is also often the case that other mental health problems often co-occur with a decline in brain function. Another point worth making is that dementia does not only affect older people there are, as Alzheimer noted, early onset cases but, in general, the figures are that 5% of the over 60s will develop dementia, more than 20% of the over 80s and over 30% of those over 95 will develop dementia (Hughes, 2013). This means that the majority of older people will not have dementia, however, as people age the risk increases significantly. As lower- and middle-income countries are predicted to see the highest rises in their ageing populations due to better survival rates into old age then it is expected that they will see the highest rates of increase in cases of dementia (ibid.). Given the high costs of dementia care this will have a profound effect on either the costs to the economies of these countries or, in those countries where money simply isn't available, the impact will be on the quality of care available.

The World Health Organization (WHO, 2017b) estimate that there are around 50 million people worldwide living with dementia and the prevalence rate is between 5–8 cases per 100 people. Early onset dementia (people under 65) accounts for around 9% of cases. Dementia is made up of a number of different conditions of which Alzheimer's makes up about 60–70 per cent of cases. During the course of Alzheimer's disease, proteins build up in the brain to form structures called 'plaques' and 'tangles'. This leads to the loss of connections between nerve cells and eventually to the death of nerve cells and loss of brain tissue. The other main types of dementia are vascular dementia, dementia with Lewy bodies (DLB) and FTD. It is possible to have more than one type of dementia (mixed dementia) which is most often Alzheimer's with vascular dementia. The WHO (2017b) describe three stages of dementia; in the early stage, which occurs gradually and so is difficult to spot, people become more forgetful, lose track of time and can become lost in familiar places. These symptoms can be so subtle that they are not far out of what any of us may experience occasionally, especially if tired or physically unwell. As dementia progresses the structure and chemistry of the brain changes. As this happens brain cells die and the brain becomes progressively more damaged. In the middle stage, the symptoms become more noticeable and people can't recall recent events or people's names, they may become lost in their own homes, begin to wander and have increasing difficulty with communication. In the late stage, people experience serious memory disturbance and have difficulty recognising friends and family, they need a great deal of care and assistance, become unaware of time and where they are. People experience a range of psychological symptoms that may include aggression, anxiety, hallucinations, depression and apathy (WHO, 2017b). They also experience changes in their behaviour including disinhibition and repeated wandering.

Many footballers have been diagnosed with dementia; in 2017 the former Liverpool player Ian St John called for leaders in the game to look after ex-professionals diagnosed with Alzheimer's.

He said several of his former team mates have the condition. One was former Liverpool teammate Geoff Strong, who won the FA Cup in 1965 alongside St John. Strong died aged 75 from Alzheimer's in 2013 while, last year, it was revealed that three members of England's 1966 World Cup squad – Martin Peters, Nobby Stiles and Ray Wilson – have also been diagnosed with it. Former West Bromwich Albion striker Jeff Astle died in 2002, aged 59. He had been diagnosed with Alzheimer's, however, a re-examination of his brain found he had died from chronic traumatic encephalopathy (CTE). It is thought this brain trauma was caused by heading footballs throughout his career. A form of CTE is *dementia pugilistica* which is often found in boxers and was once known as being 'punch drunk'. CTE is a neuro-degenerative disorder caused by trauma such as being punched often, heading heavy footballs or receiving repeated blows to the head via tackles, such as in American football. The cause of CTE, repeated trauma means it is different to classic dementia, however, as Hughes (2013) points out repeated trauma to the head can cause dementia. Though some of the changes in the brain are different to Alzheimer's disease both are associated with atrophy to the brain and neurofibrillary tangles containing the tau protein. The only reliable way at present to diagnose CTE is by a post-mortem. A study of the post-mortem brains of 12 former American footballers conducted between 2008 and 2010 (Gavett et al., 2011) showed that all 12 were showing signs of CTE. Since then, a number of current and former athletes have pledged to donate their brains to the Bedford VA Hospital for continued research into CTE. A particularly troubling case was that of Kansas City Chiefs' linebacker Jovan Belcher, a player that took many physical hits in his footballing career. Some of his former team mates (Pearlman, 2013) are certain he suffered multiple concussions and subsequently, as a consequence, headaches, memory loss and emotional lability. On 1 December 2012, after arguing with his partner he shot her then drove to work and, in front of the general manager and several coaches, shot himself dead. A subsequent post-mortem confirmed that he had CTE.

Though physicians from the ancient world, such as Galen and Aretheus of Cappadocia, wrote about mental health conditions including a chronic decline in mental faculties it has been noted (Boller & Forbes, 1998) that there is surprisingly little documentation of dementia in classical antiquity. Among the first people to study and write about dementia were the French psychiatrists Philippe Pinel (1745–1826) and Jean-Étienne Esquirol (1772–1840). Esquirol described it as a cerebral disease characterised by an impairment of sensibility which is a description we would still recognise today, however, his listed causes for dementia included, alongside progression of age and head injuries; menstrual disorders, masturbation, haemorrhoids surgery and unhappy love (ibid.) – which demonstrates that though doctors in this era were describing diseases accurately since they did not understand the causes they were still prone to ascribe their own idiosyncratic moral and religious views to them.

One of the earliest documented cases of what is strongly suspected by many to be Alzheimer's disease is that of the Anglo-Irish author and satirist Jonathan Swift (1667–1745) (ibid.) famous for *Gulliver's Travels* among other works. Indeed, in *Gulliver's Travels* Swift describes the immortal struldbruggs who, by the age of 80, can only remember those things that they learnt in their youth and middle age, the loss of one's short term memory is a very strong feature of dementia and Swift, who wrote the book when aged 59, is possibly demonstrating an insight into the condition. It has been suggested (Lorch, 2006) that one should be cautious when proposing a retrospective diagnosis over two hundred years ago in a case such as this. However, there is documentary evidence of Swift's cognitive decline, he wrote to his friends about losing his memory as he got older, he became more paranoid and disorganised in his life and his speech was affected. Furthermore, Swift eventually became unable to write at all and was very vulnerable; to protect him his friends eventually had him declared of unsound mind and memory. When he died, Swift left the majority of his fortune in his will in order to found a hospital for the mentally ill which still exists today.

One particularly worrying aspect of dementia is its often subtle and insidious onset. This is of particular concern if the affected individual holds a position of power and or influence. Politicians are no less susceptible to developing dementia than anyone else. According to Davidson (2011), three serving British prime ministers have had dementia – Ramsay MacDonald, Winston Churchill and Harold Wilson. Another worrying example he cites is that of Lord

Tweedmouth who, as First Lord of the Admiralty, gave away classified information to the German Kaiser in 1909 several years before the two countries were at war. Ramsay MacDonald was the first ever Labour party leader to become prime minister of Britain in 1924. His position in labour history is contentious given his decision in 1931 to leave the then Labour government and form a national coalition with other parties. He stood against the Labour party in the 1931 election that saw him returned to parliament as prime minister of a coalition government and the Labour party reduced to a rump of 52 seats. It was during his reign as prime minister of the National government that his mental decline began. MacDonald was known to experience periods of depression (ibid.) but his general physical robustness also declined in the early 1930s and, as part of this, came a marked decline in his mental capabilities. By 1933 he appeared at times incoherent in his speeches in the House of Commons; the decline in his memory was noticeable as was the slowing of his thoughts. With the rise of first Mussolini and then Hitler, the international political situation became ever more challenging and MacDonald was in no fit state to lead Britain during this period, he realised this and resigned in 1935. Despite leaving office his mental and physical health continued to deteriorate and he died two years later in 1937.

A famous and tragic case of early onset dementia is that of the actor Rita Hayworth. Hayworth was a very successful actor during the 1940s but, unfortunately, she developed a drinking problem associated with the stress of being a famous actor and some difficult tempestuous marriages including one to Orson Welles. Her alcohol problems took their toll on her physically but also probably prevented the recognition of her developing Alzheimer's disease at an earlier stage. She had to retire from acting in her early fifties as she could not remember her lines. She was cared for by her daughter, Yasmin Aga Khan (now the president of Alzheimer Disease International), for many years. When she died the then president, Ronald Reagan, issued a statement praising her courage and candour at letting the world know of her Alzheimer's disease. She is credited with being one of the first people in the public eye to draw attention to Alzheimer's disease and helped increase government funding for Alzheimer's research in the USA. Other more recent examples of people who have bravely spoken publically about their experiences with dementia are the British writer Terry Pratchett who spoke often about his condition and how it affected his ability to write and the American singer Glen Campbell who was also open about his diagnosis and continued to tour for a couple of years after being diagnosed, latterly with his three youngest children in his backing band.

Many actors have had dementia including, Charles Bronson, Charlton Heston, Jack Lord, Omar Sharif and Peter Falk. Falk, famous for his TV detective Columbo, from the television program of the same name, which ran from 1971 to 2003, also had a successful film career including two Oscar nominations; he developed Alzheimer's in his last years and, after one incident in which he appeared confused in public, was rarely seen publically again. Ronald Reagan, the actor turned politician who had praised Rita Hayworth's bravery was himself formally diagnosed with Alzheimer's in 1994 five years after he left office. Some have thought it may have begun while he was still president, though even his own family can't agree on this as witnessed by an argument between two of his sons. When one wrote a book in 2011 to celebrate his father's centenary in which he suggested that his father's Alzheimer's disease began while he was in office his brother hotly disputed this.

Treatments for dementia

Dementia is experienced by the individual in their social context. In the UK about two-thirds of people with dementia live in their own homes and one-third in a residential care setting, though the numbers living in residential care rises with age (Hughes, 2011). Packages of care are often set up and monitored by governmental agencies with the aim of helping the individual live as independently as possible. It is also the case in many countries that support is available for those who care for people with dementia, as this progressive illness can take both a physical and emotional toll on carers. Developing countries have had less time to develop the health and social care services needed for their ageing populations creating a considerable challenge to public health bodies (Shaji, 2009). Though in many developing countries older people are greatly respected, the traditional model of older people being cared for in multigenerational households is under strain as families become more mobile and more women enter the workforce (ibid.).

There are a limited number of drugs that lessen some of the symptoms and that may slow down the progression of the illness for some people. However, the drugs are not suitable for all types of dementia including FTD and vascular dementia. There are currently four drugs with a licence to, treat dementia. Three of the four are classified as Acetylcholinesterase Inhibitors (AChEI) and they act by inhibiting the action of an enzyme (AChE) that breaks down acetylcholine. Acetylcholine is a neurotransmitter that acts in various parts of the brain including areas that have a role in memory and attention. It is thought that by increasing synaptic acetylcholine levels this counteracts the loss of cholinergic innervation found in Alzheimer's disease (Linden, 2012). Therefore, if prescribed in the early stages of dementia they may delay cognitive decline and in some cases temporarily improve cognitive function (ibid.). Unfortunately, as these drugs treat the symptoms (loss of acetylcholine) and not the disease process they only slow the progression and are not a cure for Alzheimer's disease. The fourth drug acts on the neurotransmitter glutamate and reviews (Robinson & Keating, 2006; Matsunaga et al., 2015) have found it to be helpful in the middle and later stages of Alzheimer's disease by reducing the decline of cognition, behaviour and function. It is sometimes used in conjunction with one of the AChEI drugs. It is thought that excessive glutamate is one of the causes of the excitotoxic injury that leads to a loss of cholinergic neurons (Robinson & Keating, 2006). The drug memantine reduces glutamate-induced cell death and is thought to be neuroprotective (ibid.), however, a review of studies of the use of memantine (Matsunaga et al., 2015) found its effect size small with limited evidence of clinical benefit.

There is no cure for dementia and treatment consists of a combination of lifestyle choices including diet and exercise, reducing or stopping smoking if the person does smoke, and managing other physical ailments that can impact on dementia such as heart disease (this is especially important for people with vascular dementia). Psychological approaches include cognitive stimulation therapy (CST), reminiscence therapy, music and arts therapies and complementary therapies, for example, massages. Cognitive Stimulation Therapy is a group therapy that aims to stimulate people with dementia, each session has a theme including such activities as word games, number games and quizzes that aim to stimulate the minds of the participants in a social setting. Though dementia is a progressive condition, if people adopt a healthy lifestyle and take a combination of social and medical treatments they can still live a fulfilling and meaningful life for many years.

4

Eating Disorders

Eating disorders are very complex and include a range of conditions that can affect someone physically, psychologically and socially. The thing that many people find challenging about eating disorders is the contradiction between the fact that they are self-imposed but at the same time self-destructive and potentially fatal disorders. The three most common eating disorders are anorexia nervosa, bulimia and binge eating disorder (BED). The first mention of binge eating was in a paper by psychiatrist Albert Stunkard in 1959 but BED wasn't recognised as a separate eating disorder until its inclusion in the revised American Diagnostic and Statisitcal Manual, DSM-IV, in 2013. It doesn't have a separate category in the WHO International Classification of Diseases (ICD) codes and is collected with other conditions under the category of 'eating disorder not otherwise specified' (EDNOS). Therefore, though BED has been recognised and described by clinicians for a very long time, as a distinct category of eating disorder it is still a relatively new construct.

Eating disorders have until recently been considered to be found almost exclusively in Western or Westernised countries where 'thinness' is considered a sign of attractiveness, especially but not solely for women. They have therefore been described as 'culture bound' syndromes. However, recent studies (Smink et al., 2012) have demonstrated that eating disorders do occur in non-Western societies and among ethnic minorities. This increasing occurrence of eating disorders in non-Western societies such as Japan, China, South Africa and Chile has been associated with modernisation, globalisation and cultural transition, including a greater media exposure to Western ideas and images (ibid.). It has been argued (Cromby et al., 2013) that there was an increase in the incidence (the number of new cases in a given time frame) of eating disorders, especially anorexia nervosa, in the latter part of the twentieth century. Though it has also been suggested (Giordano, 2005) that it is unclear whether there was actually an increase or whether other factors such as demographic changes, the availability of services to detect cases and a greater public awareness of the condition have led to an increase in the numbers of people identified and subsequently diagnosed with the conditions.

Females have a much higher prevalence (the total number of cases in a population at any given time) of eating disorders than males and males tend to develop them at a later age. Incidence rates are highest for females aged from 15–19 years old (Smink et al., 2012). Males represent about eight per cent of anorexic people and 15 per cent of those with bulimia (Giordano, 2005). Prevalence rates for anorexia and bulimia vary between studies and it has been argued (Mitchison & Hay, 2014) that there are a number of reasons for this including the fact that research into eating disorders is a small but growing area of research, the assessment methods used to identify cases vary and that the vast majority of people with eating disorders do not come to the attention of clinical services. The higher prevalence among females has long been attributed to the Western ideas that associate thinness with beauty, ideas that are reinforced by a myriad of magazines, TV programmes and other social media aimed primarily at young women. Fashion models and female celebrities that are identified as exemplars of beauty are often very thin. It is also the case that young girls are subject to intense peer pressure and that, at times, this may drive them towards restricted eating. A number of robust studies have demonstrated that exposure to any of these various influences is linked to an increase in body dissatisfaction, weight concerns and weight restricting behaviours (Culbert et al., 2015). However, only a minority of young women exposed to such media images or associated pressures develop eating disorders (Cromby et al., 2013) therefore one has to be cautious about how strong the link is between societal pressures and rates of eating disorders.

As well as societal pressures to conform to certain perceptions of beauty there are other reasons why women are more prone than men to eating disorders. Societal changes have placed increasing numbers of often contradictory demands on women. Women are expected to be good mothers and good wives while at the same time be beautiful, well educated, independently minded and have careers. It has been argued that these competing pressures to be perfect both at home and successful outside the home lead to eating disorders in women who accept this concept of the 'superwoman' because it is impossible to achieve (Gordon, 1990). Furthermore, societal messages are contradictory in that they demand women be beautiful and sexual beings yet at the same time place a high value on women being so thin that they are androgynous and lacking in femininity. An inability to achieve this imagined ideal shape or make sense of the contradictions in the roles that women should aspire to are further sources of confusion and low self-esteem in women. It has been argued that eating disorders are a reaction to these societal pressures and an attempt by women to control at least one aspect of their lives (Giordano, 2005). This has been supported by the observation that eating problems usually develop around adolescence; a time in life also associated with many changes including a greater awareness of one's body and the changes that occur as adulthood approaches. The presence of an external influence or pressure shouldn't be viewed in a narrow deterministic sense as being a causal factor for an eating disorder as this ignores other factors such as self-esteem (Cromby et al., 2013) and the fact that individuals are not victims without choice or self-determination.

It has been suggested that young girls restrict their eating in an attempt to resist the onset of maturation to avoid criticism and attention from others and, in some cases, this avoidance is linked to adverse events in childhood such as sexual abuse (ibid.) – a view supported by the fact that high rates of childhood sexual abuse and other forms of childhood trauma have been found among young women with eating disorders, especially bulimia (Rayworth et al., 2004). It is surmised that some girls are attempting to avoid sexual maturation, however, as with many of the other theories about why young women develop eating disorders the relationship between external influences, internal susceptibility and subsequent behaviours is unclear.

The observation that eating disorders run in some families has stimulated studies into potential genetic factors involved in their development. Twin and adoption studies have highlighted that genetic influences contribute substantially to eating disorders (Culbert et al., 2015). Twin studies have shown a high degree of concordance especially in identical twins, however, small sample sizes make it difficult to detect the influence of shared environmental effects (Fairburn & Harrison, 2003), so actually separating out environmental from genetic factors is still to be achieved. There also seems to be cross-transmission between anorexia, bulimia and atypical eating disorders. However, the pattern of familial transmission remains unclear. Genetic association studies have concentrated on polymorphisms in serotonin related genes due to its importance in regulating eating and mood (ibid.), other neurotransmitters such as dopamine have also been studied. So far, though a genetic link seems likely, few studies that have identified a possible candidate gene have been able to replicate their findings in subsequent studies therefore the actual genetic link remains unidentified. It has been suggested (Culbert et al., 2015) that the reason why specific gene effects have not been detected is because genes act in association with environmental effects rather than independently.

Anorexia nervosa

The WHO defines anorexia nervosa as a disorder characterised by deliberate weight loss, induced and sustained by the patient. There is usually a self-perception of being too fat, an intense fear of gaining weight, or persistent behaviour that interferes with weight gain. It occurs most commonly in adolescent girls and young women, but adolescent boys and young men may also be affected. Children approaching puberty and older women up to the menopause are also affected. For some the disorder is short-lived or requires only brief interventions, however, in 10–20 per cent of cases the disorder becomes unremitting (Fairburn & Harrison, 2003). Even in cases that have responded well there are usually residual features such as continued concerns about shape, weight and eating (ibid.) (see Figure 4.1).

The term 'anorexia nervosa' was coined by the English physician William Gull in 1873 when he described a disease, mainly occurring

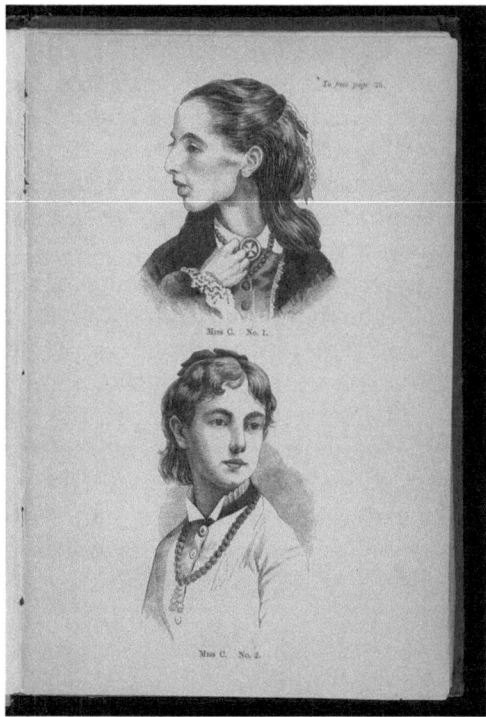

Figure 4.1 Two woodcuts showing Miss C. before and after treatment in *Anorexia Nervosa* by William Withey Gull, M.D. published in Transactions of the Clinical Society of London. (Wellcome Collection).

in young women, characterised by extreme emaciation (Jacobs Brumberg, 2000). Gull published a paper *Anorexia Nervosa* that consisted of three case studies that would be very familiar to people who have studied anorexia in modern times. Interestingly at around the same time that Gull was describing his anorexic patients the French physician Charles Lasegue published a paper entitled *De L'Anorexie Histerique*. This paper was clearly describing the same condition though with a different emphasis as Lasegue focussed more on psychological components of the disorder and family dynamics (ibid.). For Gull the disorder was caused by a diseased mental state in all probability caused by a physical neurological cause (ibid.). He paid no attention to psychological influences and recommended that patients be subject to moral control and a nutritional programme including being fed every two hours by nursing staff. In his three case studies he did treat the three young women in an individualised way, tailoring his interventions to the particular needs of each person. He did not believe they needed admission to an asylum but he did think that relatives should be kept at arm's length from the patient due to their tendency to want to indulge them.

Lasegue's explanation for anorexia was that it was a hysteria of the gastric centre. For Lasegue family dynamics were far more important in the development and maintenance of anorexia. He conceptualised anorexia as something specific to middle-class families and that the pressures on girls and young women, especially expectations that they should marry, met with resistance in the form of anorexia (ibid.). He described in detail the anxieties and various strategies of the family as they tried to encourage the anorexic person to eat. He also described how the anorexic person becomes the centre of the family's concern wielding considerable power within the family. Though Lasegue gives few details of his treatments, like Gull he indicates they were a combination of moral exhortation and nutritional encouragements to eat.

Gull's paper wasn't the first time that the condition had been described however – the English physician Richard Morton had described the case of a young woman with what he termed 'nervous consumption' in his *Treatise of Consumptions* in 1694 which would also seem familiar to contemporary eyes. The term literally means 'lack of appetite' but people with anorexia do feel hungry but they try to suppress their appetite. Food is of major importance in an anorexic's life as they, like others in a state of starvation, think constantly of food. The disorder is associated with a specific psychopathology whereby a dread of fatness and flabbiness of body contour persists as an intrusive overvalued idea, and the patients impose a low weight threshold on themselves. The symptoms include restricted dietary choice, excessive exercise, induced vomiting and purgation, and use of appetite suppressants and diuretics.

Between Morton and Gull and Lasegue lie almost 200 hundred years where physicians have talked of many hysterical and nervous conditions in women but none have really described any cases that are so clearly identifiable as anorexia as those cases described by Morton, Gull and Lasegue (Bell, 1987). Given its association with modern images of women and other societal pressures it could be assumed that anorexia is essentially a modern illness. However, Bell (ibid.) argued that one can find individual examples of anorexia further back in history. Of the 261 holy women recognised by the Roman Catholic Church as saints or otherwise holy whose lives he studied between the period 1200 and the present, in his opinion roughly a third displayed clear signs of anorexia. In this sense it can be argued that anorexia is not a modern illness but goes back hundreds of years. However, it has also been pointed out (Jacobs Brumberg, 2000) that though the behaviours of refusing food, physical over activity and a preoccupation with food may be similar across the ages, the social and cultural contexts within which people (predominantly women) have acted out these behaviours have differed greatly, hence, the reasons and motivations for disordered eating have been different in different historical epochs. In this sense, Jacobs Brumberg (ibid.) argues that anorexia nervosa, as we understand it today, emerged from the economic and social environment of the late nineteenth century. Furthermore, that it was at a time of change in the nature of the family and the role of women under capitalism. Interestingly, Jacobs Brumberg (ibid.) points out that anorexia developed before the current mass cultural preoccupation with dieting and the association between slimness and female attractiveness thus highlighting that, even if viewed as a modern illness, the contextual influences that cause it have continued to change over time.

Religious fasting and disordered eating

There is a strong connection between spirituality and purity in Western Christian thought. The fourth century saint St Jerome wrote extensively on religious matters and he encouraged an ascetic lifestyle, including fasting as a way to live a more spiritual life. By the Middle Ages it became quite common, especially for women, to associate religious piety with physical purity. Moral perfection was associated with a detachment from the physical world and fasting was one way to purify the body. Food and food production was also an area in which women in the Middle Ages had a degree of control. Control, not only over the cooking of food but also over other aspects of their lives; such as bodily functions, fertility and sexuality, as all of these could all be manipulated via abstaining from food (Bynum, 1988). A refusal to eat was, in some cases, interpreted as pious but it is also true that even as far back as the Middle Ages it was variously interpreted as the result of demonic forces, divine influence or even fraudulent and attention seeking behaviour (ibid.).

When one looks at some of the cases of extreme fasting from the Middle Ages the most famous is that of Catherine of Siena (1347–1380), she was one of those people whose restricted eating was closely associated with her religious beliefs. She had become interested in religion from childhood and she began fasting as a child (ibid.). When she was approximately 16 years old she chose to dedicate her life to the service of God and she then restricted her food and fluid intake further. Eventually, after several years, she restricted it to drinking some water, chewing bitter herbs (though not swallowing them) and taking only her communion wafer. However, she did not attribute her fasting to religious piety but described it as an 'infirmity' stating she was unable to eat.

At the age of 21 years Catherine claimed to have entered into a 'mystical marriage' with Jesus of whom she had had a vision in which he claimed he wanted to marry her and given her a ring visible only to her. Some claimed she was deluded and that her refusal to eat was a form of attempted suicide and therefore a mortal sin in the eyes of the Church. Others thought she was faking it to portray herself as more holy than she was. Some thought that her ability to survive without eating was proof of demonic possession or witchcraft. To avoid such accusations she did try to eat once a day. However this hurt her stomach so much that she was compelled to vomit whatever she had attempted to eat. She induced this vomiting by inserting fennel stalks into her stomach. This cycle of eating and vomiting is very common to anorexics. Catherine described her behaviour in religious terms stating that her vomiting was penance for her sins and, indeed, in the Christian tradition fasting is seen a pious and would have been seen as especially so in the Middle Ages. This eating and vomitting went on for approximately six years according to the testimony of Raymond, her confessor, and over time she became increasingly unable to take sustenance. From early 1380 she could no longer eat or drink water, and died at the age of 33 in April 1380. What is interesting is that even then, in the fourteenth century, opinions varied widely on the cause and motives for her behaviour – whereas some saw her behaviour motivated by her love of God, others attributed baser motives to her or even the influence of demonic supernatural forces.

Bynum (ibid.) argues that in the cultural context of the Middle Ages men and women's inability, or refusal, to eat was interpreted differently. In general, women's illnesses were more likely to be seen as things to be endured not cured. In fact, as the sin of gluttony was seen as worse in women, for a woman to not eat was not seen as something needing to be cured. Furthermore, the patient suffering of an illness was seen as a significant way of gaining sanctity for females but not for males (ibid.). The increase in the numbers of women practising abstinence in the later Middle Ages was part of a wider trend in this period for the occurrence of other miraculous phenomena happening to women such as stigmata, body elongation and sweet smelling bodies. Bynum (ibid.) also argues that, though there are differences with the modern conception of anorexia as a pursuit of thinness and its equation with beauty, if one applies the psychiatrist Bruch's definition of anorexia as self-inflicted starvation in the absence of an identifiable organic cause while in the presence of ample food and also acknowledges that some of these women also displayed other symptoms that are common to modern day anorexia such as over activity and a lack of a need for sleep, then one can cautiously see considerable similarities between their condition and modern day anorexia. One cautionary note is that apart from Catherine of Siena and a few others, such as Lidwina of Schiedam (1380–1433), the historical record is quite scant and in some cases it is recorded through the prism of religious zeal which leaves its accuracy open to question.

Lidwina was a Dutch girl from the town of Schiedam. At 15 years old she became ill and several weeks later had a fall while ice skating, during which she suffered internal injuries. She is now the patron saint of ice skaters, as well as the chronically ill, and of the town of

Schiedam. After her accident she became paralysed except for her left hand and her body putrefied with bits of it falling off and, as if this wasn't enough, blood poured from her ears, nose and mouth. Also at this time she began to fast. After a while she ate nothing and only drank half a pint of watered wine per week. She became famous locally for her holiness and it was claimed that her bodily emissions cured other people; though others suspected that her fasts, too, were a sign of demonic possession. She apparently shed skin, bones and parts of her intestines (ibid.) which gave off a sweet-smelling odour. Her local town officials had her watched and produced a document stating that she was observed not to eat for three full months. She eventually died at the age of 53.

Fasting girls

As we have seen, opinions on a refusal to eat have always varied, while some saw it as a sign of holiness others saw it as a sign of demonic possession or as pure fakery. As Europe changed with the rise of Protestantism and the Reformation, such extravagant signs of holiness became less acceptable. However, this does not mean that disordered eating disappeared, only that it's perception and status changed. The phenomenon of 'fasting girls' has many parallels with modern anorexia in that it occurred usually in teenage girls or young women who refused to eat and who said that eating made them feel ill. Some of their stories also had religious elements but, in general, they were less intensely religious in character than the earlier Middle Age mystics. Often, like Lidwina, the trigger for their refusal to eat was some accident or illness: Martha Taylor, the so-called 'Derbyshire Damsel', began her fast in 1667 some time after receiving a blow to the back; Mollie Fancher (1848–1916) was involved in two accidents and shortly after the second one took to her bed and stated she could live without food; and Sarah Jacob (1857–1869) had some kind of convulsions at the age of nine years, after which she too took to her bed and refused food. There are other similarities in these cases, all three became local celebrities as news of their ability to live without food spread, for those that believed them they were seen as miraculous, and for many they were thought to be frauds and were subjected to close scrutiny.

Martha Taylor, a 19-year-old from Over-Haddon in Derbyshire, claimed she refused to eat food from December 1667. She became the subject of several pamphlets (Jacobs Brumberg, 2000) over the next few years with titles such as *Newes from Derbyshire,* or the *Wonder of all Wonders, The Wonder of the World* and *A discourse of prodigious abstinence, occasioned by the twelve months fasting of Martha Taylor,* the last of which went for a less hyperbolic and more descriptive title. Despite claims that she had not eaten for two years her face was described in one of the pamphlets as 'plump and ruddy'. Unlike other famous cases, Martha Taylor seems to have passed from history as little is known of what happened to her after 1669.

The case of Sarah Jacobs did not have such an unremarkable ending, unfortunately for her. Sarah grew up in Carmarthenshire, Wales, and began to fast at the age of 12. Her parents claimed she had eaten nothing since October 1867 but, despite this, she looked well and seemed to thrive. It's also clear that the locals in her village believed her and she became a local celebrity. Her fame spread even further when her local vicar, the Reverend Jones, wrote to the newspapers and her fasting became known much further afield. This was to have tragic consequences for Sarah. People began to visit her from all over Wales and from further afield including England, walking over 2 miles from the nearest train station to the farm where she lived. In early 1869 she was subjected to a 24-hour watch for 2 weeks and was declared genuine, as the two men watching over her in shifts never saw her eat. The controversy of the authenticity of her fasting did not go away however, and a committee of concerned locals wrote to the London medical establishment in November 1869 to ask for their help in settling the matter (ibid.).

Four nurses were dispatched from Guy's Hospital to organise the watch. The rooms of the house were searched for food, her room was prepared including asking that her sister no longer sleep with her and that her parents' bed be removed from her room to better control the environment under watch. According to the later court report of the case, when the nurses arrived she was still 'a fine, plump handsome child' (*Tivyside Advertiser,* 1870). Sarah's parents informed the nurses that being urged to eat made their daughter worse so they should not offer her food (Jacobs Brumberg, 2000). Now, to us, it is clear that Sarah could not have lived for two years without food and must have been surviving somehow by eating and drinking clandestinely, which makes it strange that her parents were so forceful in their statements that no help should be offered to their daughter. In the first couple of days the nurses observed a urine and faeces stained nightdress indicating she had been taking nourishment.

Over the next few days however Sarah became increasingly weaker. The nurses appealed to the doctors and the parents to end the observations so that Sarah could recommence taking nourishment by whatever means, the doctors agreed, the parents did not. Therefore the experiment, for that is what it had become, continued and on the tenth day Sarah Jacobs died of starvation. During this time both the doctors and nurses from London, and the Jacobs' own family doctor, advised calling off the experiment but the parents continued to refuse despite their daughter's noticeable deterioration (ibid.). Even though all parties were culpable by continuing with the experiment and not offering Sarah any food or fluid, the medical staff were discharged from blame but her parents were later found guilty of manslaughter. Tragically, at her post-mortem, there were signs on her body such as an indentation under her right arm similar in shape to a half pint bottle and some small bones in her stomach that indicated that, prior to the watch, she had been taking some form of sustenance. Why then were her parents so forceful in their arguments that no food be offered to their daughter? Maybe on one level they grew to believe the story themselves. It is also true that they were poor farmers and their daughter's fame brought money and gifts that made their lives easier, indeed the newspaper report of their trial describes them as 'reduced to the extremest poverty' (*Tivyside Advertiser*, 1870) after the tragic death of their daughter. The Sarah Jacob's case, and others like it, provided the material for the novel *The Wonder* by Emma Donoghue which treats the subject in a sensitive and exciting manner.

At a similar time to Sarah Jacob a young woman named Mollie Fancher became known as the 'Brooklyn Enigma' in the USA (Jacobs Brumberg, 2000). She initially became ill with what was described as nervous indigestion which left her with an inability to eat. The later accidents mentioned above triggered a strange array of symptoms including periodic blindness and deafness. She took to her bed and became an invalid, losing the use of her legs and one arm. She also claimed to have some other supernatural powers, such as being able to see into the future and read a book just by passing her hand over its cover. Over time she claimed to have lived off practically no food for 14 years. She was described as emaciated and was never observed to eat. People, especially members of the New York Neurological Society such as William Hammond, wanted to test whether she was truly fasting or cheating, he was convinced that she was just another 'hysterical' woman and was eating in secret (ibid.). However, people were wary of repeating what had happened to Sarah Jacob several years before as knowledge of that case had spread to the USA and other parts of the world. Hammond and other medical men tried to goad Fancher into demonstrating her powers via pieces in local papers, but she wisely ignored them. It is easy to understand the exasperation of men such as Hammond. Committed as they were to the growing discipline of science, they were moving away from religious and supernatural explanations of the world. They must have found it hard to believe that a woman could claim to exist without eating for many years and be able to foretell the future and, even harder to understand, was that many people believed her.

The explanation given by the medical men for the behaviour of Fancher (for all the contemporary opinions I have seen proffered were by men) was the norm for a woman describing a range of physical and emotional symptoms, namely hysteria. For late-nineteenth century medical men, the fact that Fancher was bedridden supported their view that she would require only minimal food and fluids. The fact that she was female meant, therefore, that she was a hysteric, acting as she did to gain attention, and in their view was emotionally immature and deceitful. Hysteria was an explanation for anorexia also supported by Freud and other psychoanalysts. They saw, in the refusal of food and its associated symptoms including amenorrhoea and a lack of adult female curves, a refusal by the anorexic of adult female sexuality (ibid.). The Fancher case continued to cause controversy and argument between various members of the medical profession for many years. Fancher herself lived well into her 60s and died in 1916 shortly after spending 50 years in her bed.

The development of the modern conception of anorexia

During the period covering the end of the nineteenth and into the first decades of the twentieth century the emphasis on thinness, especially for females, was associated with social class since a thinner, almost frail, physique identified a woman as too weak for work and obviously of a higher social status than working women (ibid.). It was also an era where dieting became more popular and was advertised frequently in the mainstream newspapers and magazines of the day, indeed, even cigarettes were advertised to women as an alternative to food to encourage them to avoid putting on weight. However, in general, anorexia was only known to medical professionals and didn't really enter into the public consciousness until the 1960s (Appignanesi, 2009). In the early part of the twentieth century two distinct approaches to treating anorexics, the biological and the psychoanalytical, developed. Psychoanalytical theory, as expressed by Pierre Janet, did see anorexia as a way of the person exerting some control in their life, whereas Freud saw anorexia not as a way of controlling weight but as a consequence of disgust for food which he associated with repressed sexuality (Jacobs Brumberg, 2000). Both schools, however, did see it as a behavioural manifestation of deeper underlying emotional conflicts (ibid.). The biological approach focussed on various organs, such as the pituitary and the thyroid glands, which were thought to be faulty and so patients were injected with glandular extracts to replace the supposed insufficiency. The problem with injecting thyroid hormones was that it increased metabolic activity and, therefore, would increase weight loss so it was vital that the patients were also fed a highly nutritious diet.

An influential figure in widening the discussion about the causes and treatments of anorexia was the German Jewish doctor Hilde Bruch, who had fled Nazi Germany in 1933 and settled in the US. In her book entitled *Eating Disorders* she drew heavily on her psycho-analytical training and experience. She was at pains not to medical-ise people with eating disorders but spoke about the role that food plays in the family as a means of rewarding and punishing children. Bruch (1973) thought that the roots of eating disorders went back to the person's earliest experiences as a child. She also discussed the

complex roles that food plays in all human societies and linked anorexia to obesity, stating that both are related to faulty hunger awareness. She also stressed that both are complex conditions that cannot
be explained by one simple mechanism but that they develop as an
expression of a disturbance in the interaction between physiochemi-
cal, physiological, psychological and social factors. In this sense
Bruch was integrating the biological and psychological perspectives
into a complex unitary system (ibid.). Bruch was writing at a time of
great social change, an era more receptive to complex explanations of
phenomena such as eating disorders. At the same time others coming from the feminist movement, such as the psychotherapist Susie
Orbach and the writer Germaine Greer also addressed eating disorders and sought to place them within the context of a male-domi-
nated society that places many competing, and often contradictory,
demands on young girls and women.

There are many books by survivors of anorexia that detail each
individual's unique struggle with eating and what has helped them
to overcome it (if indeed they have). Sadly, some people succumb to
anorexia, a famous example of this is the singer and drummer Karen
Carpenter (1950–1983). She formed a very successful pop group with
her brother Richard. As she was only 5 feet 4 inches tall it was difficult
for audiences to see her singing behind her drum kit so, as the band
became more successful, they recruited other drummers so that Karen
could stand up front with a microphone and been seen. It appears
that Karen became concerned about her weight at college in the mid-
1960s, not long after starting her first group with her brother Richard
while she was still at high school. As the group became successful
they embarked on a gruelling touring schedule that took its toll on
both Karen and Richard. Richard became addicted to the sedative,
methaqualone, and Karen's concerns about her weight tipped over
into anorexia and her weight plummeted. The group began cancelling
appearances by the mid-1970s and by 1978 neither of them was in a
fit state to tour; in 1979 Richard entered treatment to address his
addiction.

Though Richard recovered from his addiction after a period in
rehab, Karen continued to suffer from anorexia. She tried to continue
working and there is a lot of footage of her being interviewed or
performing in which she is obviously very underweight despite

her attempts to hide it with loose fitting and/or multiple layers of clothes. The stress of being in a successful act was accentuated by personal problems, Karen felt unloved by her mother and experienced low self-esteem – choosing how much she ate was one of the few areas in her life where she still felt in control (Schmidt, 2011). By 1980, Karen had met and married a real-estate developer. Unfortunately, he had not disclosed the fact that he had had a vasectomy and, as Karen wanted children, this was shocking news. It has been reported (ibid.) that Karen tried to call off the wedding but her mother wouldn't let her do it. Soon after they were married it became apparent that he was also far less well off financially than he had led Karen to believe. This led to the failure of her marriage. With her personal life at such a low Karen attempted to regain control of her anorexia by seeking therapy in New York from Steven Levenkron, a psychotherapist who had recently written a highly successful novel about eating disorders called *The Best Little Girl in the World*. By this time Karen was abusing laxatives and thyroid medication (it speeds up the metabolism) to enhance her weight loss. She also continued to exercise a lot and to walk to her therapy sessions. Unfortunately, Karen continued to deteriorate and was hospitalised in New York in September 1982. In hospital she was fed intravenously due to her low weight and dehydration. She quickly regained some weight and, having decided the therapy in New York wasn't working, returned to California in November 1982. Unfortunately, she deteriorated again and died in early February 1993. The cause of death was 'emetine cardiotoxicity due to or as a consequence of anorexia nervosa'. Emetine is also known as Ipecac an emetic used to induce vomiting. She was 32 years old.

Unfortunately, many people succumb to anorexia and, unsurprisingly given the pressure to be excessively thin, a number of fashion models are among them. Tragically, among their number are the sisters Luisel and Eliana Ramos who both died of heart failure caused by anorexia only several months apart. Some people believe that the Scottish child star Lena Zavaroni died from her anorexia; however she also suffered from depression and was so desperate to be free of her depressive illness that she underwent psychosurgery. Initially it seemed to be successful but, unfortunately, she contracted bronchial pneumonia and died 3 weeks later aged 35. Michael Krasnow, the author who wrote the book *My Life as a Male Anorexic*, died at the age of 28. Krasnow's book is not just a description of his experiences of anorexia, he also details how he believes the medical industry in the USA failed him. Krasnow was a perfectionist and hated the demands to gain weight that many of his doctors made on him, in fact some eating disorder specialists refused to treat him until he reached a specific weight. However, as he was unlikely to want to gain weight without specialist help, this paradoxically meant this help was denied him. This battle of wills defined much of his contact with the medical services. After a number of compulsory admissions to hospital and episodes of force-feeding he moved away and, despite a very low weight, was able to work in his uncle's finance company. Eventually his body could no longer function at the near-starvation weight he tried to maintain and his mother found him one morning, dead in his apartment.

With help many people do recover from anorexia. Most patients recover within five years and most relapses occur in the first two years after treatment, often when the individual is subject to stressful situations (Abraham, 2016). However, it is also true that there is no empirically supported treatment of choice for all patients and treatment is also made more difficult by the fact that many people with anorexia do not think it is a 'problem' and hence refuse treatment (Steinglass et al., 2016). Despite this, there are numerous examples of people who have experienced anorexia and recovered to varying degrees. This is supported by the number of people who have been open about their eating disorders and what they found helpful in overcoming them, including the model Kate Dillon Levin, the actresses Jane Fonda, Felicity Huffman, Portia de Rossi and Calista Flockhart, and the singers Melanie Chisholm and Alanis Morissette. Huffman has stated she suffered from both anorexia and bulimia in her 20s and the unconditional love and acceptance she received from her husband, the fellow actor William H. Macy, helped to convince her that she didn't need to be a different body shape to be accepted. Chisholm found the attention that came with the fame of being one of the Spice Girls difficult to cope with and suffered with various forms of eating disorders; she has said that a combination of factors including therapy, counselling, alternative therapy and acupuncture all helped her.

Treatment approaches to anorexia

Given the complexities of anorexia, the individual reasons why people develop it, the severity of it and the methods employed to restrict eating, it should be no surprise that different interventions work for different people and to different extents. Unfortunately, for some people nothing seems to be effective. The best treatment approaches are those that are collaborative where the person with anorexia engages with the therapy.

Various talking therapies have been demonstrated to be effective with anorexia though it has been pointed out (Abraham, 2016) that, at a very low body weight, psychological treatment is of limited value as the person will find it difficult to concentrate and will lack the energy to engage in the therapeutic process. Patients will be experiencing both the physical weakness associated with starvation and the psychological effects, such as poor concentration and an internal focus on their eating and weight, will make it impossible to engage in any meaningful way with therapy. Therefore, if the individual is of such a low body weight then medical stabilisation will be necessary before any psychological treatment can begin. Indeed, if their weight is so low that it threatens to lead to organ failure or even death, then the first goal is to treat this medical emergency. This may mean admission to a general hospital if their weight is so low that assisted feeding is necessary. This could also mean legally detaining an individual and feeding them against their will via a nasogastric tube. This is very invasive and, as it takes the responsibility for eating away from the individual and does not teach them 'normal' eating behaviour (ibid.), it should usually only be used as a last resort.

Attempts to treat anorexia with medication have not yielded positive results. Given the association with depressive and anxiety type symptoms, antidepressants are a class of drug that have been among the most widely studied. Unfortunately, no trials have demonstrated the efficacy of antidepressants. Similarly, drugs used to treat anxiety (anxiolytics) have also failed to show any impact on eating behaviour. There is a long history of studies using antipsychotics to try to treat anorexia, and evidence (Steinglass et al., 2016) seems to suggest that some of the newer antipsychotics may be effective in treating some of the obsessive ruminations that accompany anorexia.

However, antipsychotics and some classes of antidepressants can affect an individual's heart so, if the individual is of a very low weight, it is likely that their heart is already under strain and such medication should be avoided.

Of the various therapy options available Bruch advocated family therapy, seeing the causes of anorexia in family dynamics. Modern approaches to family-based therapy encourage participation by the whole family and are used mostly with younger people. There are various forms of family therapy but they all tend to be offered on an outpatient basis. Other therapies that are used to treat anorexia include cognitive analytic therapy (CAT), interpersonal psychotherapy (IPT) and CBT. The evidence base for IPT with anorexia is weak and even proponents of its use with bulimia (where it will be discussed more fully) do not recommend it for anorexia (Murphy et al., 2012).

All the talking therapies can be offered in a range of settings from individual therapists through to eating disorder services that offer therapy and interventions. CBT is recommended in the UK by the National Institute for Health and Care Excellence (NICE, 2017). In therapy, CBT initially focusses on psycho-education identifying the medical and psychological effects of being underweight. The individual is encouraged to identify the beliefs that have placed a value on being low in weight, beliefs that may have been generated by issues with low self-esteem. Alongside efforts to change restrictive eating behaviours, CBT attempts to challenge these 'faulty' beliefs about eating, weight and body shape. Like other talking therapies though, CBT is usually offered to individuals above a certain body mass index to ensure that they are likely to be able to engage in therapy. This means, however, that the evidence base for its and other psychological therapies' effectiveness in treating low weight anorexia patients is lacking (Fairburn & Harrison, 2003).

Bulimia nervosa

Bulimia nervosa is the act of controlling one's weight by bingeing and then purging food, and it has ancient origins. It can be seen as an attempt to control weight that results in a loss of control and

Appignanesi (2009) states that people with bulimia are not the saints of the eating disorders community but the impulsive sinners. Supporting this view of impulsivity Casper (1983) describes the person with bulimia nervosa as psychologically different from the person with anorexia, as they have more affective impulsivity and greater impulse dyscontrol. The word bulimia comes from the Greek and literally means 'ravenous hunger'. Ancient Egyptian physicians recommended periodical purgation as a health practice. In ancient Rome people were known to induce vomiting to purge themselves after a large meal. This wasn't necessarily driven by the same morbid dread of fatness that is a core component of modern day bulimia nervosa since individuals, such as the Roman Emperor Claudius, were both obese and known to purge. However, similar to today, the purging was used as a way of preventing the overeating leading to further weight gain.

Bulimia nervosa was first used as a term in a paper by Professor Gerald Russell in 1979 and was described has having close links to anorexia in that they both stem from the same psychopathology. Russell (1979) saw bulimia nervosa as a new disorder arising out of anorexia nervosa. The condition was described as having three core components and, unlike many psychiatric diagnoses, has changed little since it was first described. The three components are: first, episodic overeating coupled with a preoccupation with food and a craving for it; second, attempts to counteract the overeating by strategies including vomiting, using medication such as appetite suppressants, diuretics, thyroids preparations and laxatives; and third, the person has a morbid fear of fatness.

Russell (1997) suggested that, with such a specific clinical description, it would be very difficult to find historical examples of bulimia. Furthermore, he argued that, unlike anorexia, bulimia nervosa is a more modern contemporary illness. Russell (ibid.) stated that accounts of overeating or vomiting in ancient literature do not equate to the modern disorder of bulimia nervosa. He therefore argued that accounts from ancient historic literature are unhelpful when discussing the modern phenomenon of bulimia nervosa. Russell (ibid.), when discussing accounts of bingeing and purging such as those of Claudius and other cases from antiquity, pointed out that Claudius and others were often also obese and do not appear to satisfy the third criteria of a morbid fear of fatness and, therefore, do not fit the diagnostic criteria for bulimia nervosa.

In fact Russell (ibid.), having reviewed studies that looked for earlier examples of bulimia nervosa and found none that included all three diagnostic criteria, argued that bulimia nervosa is essentially a disease that arises in the twentieth century and ancient examples of bingeing or purging, or even combinations of both bingeing and purging, lack the association with the dread of fatness that is key to the diagnosis. To support this, Russell describes several clinical cases of what he sees as convincing forerunners of bulimia nervosa the earliest of which 'Nadia' dates to 1903. Having said that, he does accept that certain historical figures such as the catholic saints Saint Mary Magdalene de' Pazzi (1566–1607) and Saint Veronica (1660–1727) both exhibited bulimic behaviours though he states that their binge eating and vomiting was an occasional feature of their abstinence from food and that they should more correctly be viewed as anorexics.

In recent years, more and more people have felt comfortable in coming forward to share their struggles with their weight and body shape, and that part of these struggles has been bulimia. One person that has spoken candidly about it is the American actress and political activist Jane Fonda; she has said that she suffered from bulimia for 25 years. This was triggered in childhood by her father Henry Fonda's comments that looks were vitally important to success and his critical comments of her made Fonda very insecure. She has said that she started to recover when she started her exercise workout programme and felt that she was empowering herself. She also took an antidepressant, fluoxetine, which she has said helped with her anxiety. Appignanesi (2009) has highlighted that the condition allows for a controlled pleasingly thin façade and that bulimics often continue to function well in work and personal relationships. Therefore it has included, like Fonda, a number of other famous individuals including Princess Diana, about whom much has been written. Another successful person is the American actress Diane Keaton; she has talked about the obsessive quality of bulimia and how obsessed she became with food. Also, that she was able to conceal it from her, then partner, Woody Allen. This also demonstrates the secretive nature of the disorder and the degree of shame that many sufferers experience.

Keaton has said that her insecurity and anxiety led Allen to advise her to see a psychoanalyst which subsequently helped her recover.

There have also been a number of males that have spoken about their bulimia including the former Formula One racing driver David Coulthard, the singer Elton John and the British politician John Prescott. Elton John had at one point lost control of many aspects of his life, he was drinking alcohol excessively, he was taking lots of illicit drugs and his eating had also become disordered. He has said that he would go three days without eating then gorge on sandwiches and ice cream. He attributes this to his low self-esteem and the difficulties that accompanied his fame. He recovered with a combination of rehab for his addictions and therapy for his mental health issues, including his bulimia.

Treatment of bulimia

Treatments for bulimia have been demonstrated to be effective. Though, with estimates of 80 per cent of people recovered or improved from 10–15 years after treatment (Abraham, 2016), there are still a significant number of people who continue to suffer from the condition. A review of over 50 randomised controlled trials (Fairburn & Harrison, 2003) found three robust findings from the literature: first, that a specifically designed type of CBT was the most effective therapy; second, that antidepressant drugs are also effective; and third, that, unfortunately, no consistent predictors of outcome have been identified. Various classes of antidepressants have been demonstrated to be effective for bulimia nervosa, however the most extensively studied group were the selective serotonin reuptake inhibitors (SSRIs) and all treatment guidelines recommend their use due to their tolerability and efficacy. Fairburn and Harrison (ibid.) also found weaker evidence to suggest that combining antidepressants with CBT resulted in few consistent benefits over CBT alone.

The model of CBT designed specifically to treat bulimia is a manualised therapy that focusses initially on the attitudes and beliefs of the individual, especially maladaptive assumptions about the importance of weight and shape. These assumptions lead to maladaptive behaviours such as binge eating and purging. The therapy usually involves around twenty sessions and research (ibid.) suggests that between a third to a half of those that engage with the therapy make a full recovery. Research into another type of therapy, IPT, has demonstrated that it performs well for bulimia but a comparison of it to CBT found CBT to be superior (Agras et al., 2000) both in the percentage of people that improved and also that people improved more rapidly with CBT and needed far fewer sessions.

Interpersonal psychotherapy seeks to help the individual make interpersonal changes in areas that have been identified as problematic. Relationship difficulties are common in people with eating disorders and are often a maintaining factor. IPT is a therapy that is designed to work indirectly on the eating disorder by individuals making significant interpersonal changes. It is hoped that by improving their interpersonal life this will have a positive effect on how individuals evaluate themselves. This improvement in self-esteem can then have a positive effect on eating disorder behaviour (Murphy et al., 2012). People undertaking therapy are encouraged to maintain their usual activities such as employment. The therapy is highly structured comprising 16–20 sessions of 50 minutes structured over three distinct phases. As there have been fewer studies into its effectiveness than there have been for CBT there is still a need for more research to fully assess its relative efficacy compared to CBT.

As we have seen, eating disorders have a long history in human societies. They are often embedded in cultural views of beauty and people, especially women, can feel the pressure of societal expectations of how they should look. This may seem counter-intuitive at the present time, where rates of obesity have increased significantly in a generation. However, no society lives in a monoculture where only one view has sway over what people think. This is why we can have super-thin models; increasing use of steroids, especially by males, to bulk up and obesity all within the same society. The reasons for all of these are complex and multifactorial. Fortunately, there are increasing debates in societies across the world about these issues which will hopefully aid understanding. In the field of eating disorders there is a growing body of evidence that some forms of talking therapy and, in some cases, medication are effective in treating these very serious and complex disorders.

5

Psychosis

Psychotic symptoms are as old as humanity. The way these experiences have been understood by the person experiencing them, and how they have been explained by the wider society within which these people have lived, has changed throughout the course of human history. It would be wrong and over simplistic, though, to state that at a certain point in time such symptoms as hearing a voice when there is no one around (now commonly described as auditory hallucinations) or seeing things that other people cannot see (now commonly described as visual hallucinations) were understood in a certain way and that how they have been understood has changed in different historical periods. At certain points in history different groups in different parts of the word have generated significantly different explanations influenced by the local cultural, political and religious milieu that they lived in for these experiences. This remains true to this day, in fact it is true that even within cultures the origins, meanings and even the best approaches to deal with psychotic symptoms generate fierce debate. A good example of this is the current split between two camps within Western mental health services. Crudely, this splits down the lines of two disciplines; psychiatrists and psychologists. However, even within the two disciplines there are considerable disagreements and so the actual picture is far more complex than some of the protagonists would have people believe. But protagonists some of the parties are. Within psychiatry there are those psychiatrists who believe that psychosis is essentially a brain disorder and that research into treatments should focus largely on medication and other physical treatments for the disorder. It would be wrong, though, to characterise all psychiatrists as 'biological' psychiatrists as many are also interested in the social and psychological aspects of the illness. Opposed to the biological psychiatrists are those psychologists that argue that the usual diagnostic label for people with long term psychotic illnesses (schizophrenia) is invalid and essentially meaningless. They argue that schizophrenia is such a broad catch-all label, encompassing a vast array of potential symptoms, to make it meaningless in strict diagnostic terms. They propose not treating people along diagnostic lines but in response to the symptoms they present with. They are also often hostile to 'biological' treatments such as medication (Bentall & Morrison, 2002) questioning how effective they are and arguing that non-medical treatments, such as talking therapies, should be used not in conjunction with medication but in place of them.

Throughout this chapter, I will use the terms 'schizophrenia' and 'psychosis' interchangeably – however, it is important to note that, though all psychotic symptoms can be symptoms of schizophrenia, people with schizophrenia may also experience symptoms other than psychotic symptoms. Symptoms such as low mood, a lack of volition and social withdrawal are also often part of the clinical picture with which people present. Also, it's equally true that people may experience psychotic or quasi-psychotic symptoms and not attract the diagnosis of schizophrenia. A number of researchers have pointed out that symptoms such as hearing voices are actually quite common. A number of studies of students have consistently found that around 37–39 per cent report experiencing hearing voices and general population studies have found rates of between 10 and 25 per cent of people who have experienced hearing voices at least once (Morrison et al., 2000).

Schizophrenia is a complex disorder characterised by an array of symptoms that vary between individuals leading to diverse symptom profiles. Symptoms such as delusions (a false or erroneous belief), hallucinations and thought disorder (disorganised thinking), are often described as positive symptoms whereas other symptoms such as cognitive deficits and poverty of speech are usually described as negative symptoms (Egan & Weinberger, 1997; Harrison, 1999). Despite over a hundred years of refinements in the description of schizophrenia, its classification has never been free of controversy, as each subsequent generation of psychiatrists and psychologists has challenged the conceptual framework used by the previous generation and sought to change its parameters.

Psychiatrists in the nineteenth century were inspired by advances in general medicine where clinically identifiable syndromes were being described, and sought to replicate this for the existing global concepts of dementia, delirium and insanity (Wing & Agrawal, 2003). Emile Kraepelin originally argued that dementia praecox (an early description of what later became known as schizophrenia) and manic-depressive psychosis (what we now call bipolar affective disorder) were separate entities and he was the first to systematically describe the main symptoms of each. However, Kraepelin's views were not rigid and he continued to develop them to the point that, by 1920, he came to believe that dementia praecox and manic-depressive psychosis could coexist, possibly as a unitary psychosis. Kraepelin used the term *dementia praecox* to describe psychotic illness because he believed the nature of the illness was degenerative – a dementia-like brain disease that begins in late adolescence or early adulthood with a chronic course and poor prognosis. A contemporary of Kraepelin, the Swiss psychiatrist Eugene Bleuler (1911), challenged the view that all onsets commenced in young adulthood and that degeneration occurred in all cases. He was the first to use the term *schizophrenia* as he believed that an integral component of the disorder was that different facets of mental life such as perception, thought and emotion were split off from each other. His main concern was with cognitive processes and he believed that the primary symptoms were loosening of association, affectivity, ambivalence and autism, relegating hallucinations and delusions to the status of accessory or secondary symptoms.

Bleuler (ibid.) included a much broader classification by introducing the concepts of 'simple' and 'latent' schizophrenia which both had vaguely defined primary symptoms in the absence of hallucinations and delusions. Numerous attempts have been made to identify distinct syndromes of schizophrenia; Bleuler (ibid.) subdivided schizophrenia into paranoid, hebephrenic, catatonic and simple. However, many patients have characteristics of more than one of these subtypes. Attempting to overcome the heterogeneity inherent in the concept of schizophrenia, Liddle and Barnes (1990) focused on a homogenously chronic group and identified three syndromes within this group: psychomotor poverty syndrome; disorganisation syndrome; and reality distortion syndrome. They found segregation of symptoms into one of the three syndromes possible but not entirely clear cut and, though the three syndromes were partially congruent with Bleuler's (1911) four subdivisions rather than being discrete, Liddle and Barnes (1990) asserted that all three could coexist within the same individual.

It has been argued (Bentall, 1999) that neither Kraepelin nor Bleuler regarded two very important symptoms, hallucinations and delusions, as core characteristics of schizophrenia, although they did describe them alongside other symptoms; such as thought disorder, blunted affect and lack of insight. The importance of hallucinations and delusions was shown by the work of two other psychiatrists, Karl Jaspers and Kurt Schneider, who sought to overcome the vague generalities still inherent in the concept of schizophrenia and to elucidate a clearer more specific set of symptoms. In the period from 1921 to 1955 Jaspers and Schneider developed a clear conceptualisation of delusions as ideas based on irreducible experiences not comprehensible in terms of an individual's usual attitudes and beliefs. Schneider attempted to define schizophrenia more precisely and differentiate it from manic-depressive psychosis by the development of the concept of first-rank symptoms. Schneider identified eleven first-rank symptoms which were further subdivided under the headings of hallucinations, which included auditory and visual hallucinations; delusions, which included paranoid and grandiose delusions and passivity experiences, wherein the individual believes movements, emotions or will are under the control of an external force.

The development of the concept of schizophrenia continues to be an ongoing process as current and future research will continue to challenge its conceptualisation and will lead to further revisions. However, population studies have shown that when a narrow definition relying on first-rank symptoms is used, incidence rates for schizophrenia across countries are similar and that approximately 1 per cent of a population will suffer from a schizophrenic illness (Jablensky et al., 1992). The 1992 WHO ten-country study found a narrow range of variation of incidence rates (0.16–0.42 per 1000) (Jablensky, 2003). Furthermore, a review (ibid.) of prevalence studies identified prevalence figures in the range of 1.4–4.6 per 1000 and noted that, given the differing methodologies used in these studies, this range of prevalence was quite narrow. However, this does not mean that unique psychotic syndromes in different cultures do not exist. A good example is *kitsunetsuki,* which is unique to Japanese society and occurs when the individual believes they are possessed by a fox. Other examples of culture-bound syndromes include *koro* (experienced by Chinese patients) and *latah* (experienced by Indonesians) that involve specific delusional experiences only found within their own cultural group (Bentall, 2004). Some studies, including WHO studies, have shown that people with psychosis from poorer, less well-developed societies actually do better in the long-term than people from industrialised Western societies. Unfortunately, a combination of criticisms of the research methodologies of the studies and difficulties in comparing the wide varieties of societal and cultural influences in both developed and less well-developed societies make it very difficult to draw any conclusions as to why these differences are found so often in studies. One example is that it is often found that people in developing countries with schizophrenia are more likely to be in work, however, this simple fact hides a complex picture, for example work patterns tend to be more flexible in developing counties and welfare and unemployment benefits may be non-existent meaning that people, no matter how ill, have no choice but to find some form of employment. Such factors make 'like with like' comparisons very difficult.

There are some clear gender differences in the expression of schizophrenia, for example, schizophrenia tends to occur earlier in men and they relapse more frequently (Gold, 1998). Men have been found to have higher rates of negative symptoms (Shtasel et al., 1992) and women have been found to have better outcomes in social functioning (Breier et al., 1992; Shtasel et al., 1992). Paradoxically, though, Rector and Seeman (1992) found women more likely to report auditory hallucinations, which one would expect to have a significant impact on social functioning. It has been reported (Salokangas, 2004) that men tend to be prescribed higher daily doses of antipsychotic medication. However, it has been pointed out (Gold, 1998) that men also tend to be more aggressive, a factor that is known to influence prescribing practices. Most studies (Breier et al., 1992; Gold, 1998; Salokangas, 2004) agree that further research into the complex interplay between social influences and physiological differences between the sexes is needed to explain the reasons for the differences in the expression of schizophrenia.

What causes psychotic experiences is still a matter of debate with numerous causal factors proposed. One model is the neurodevelopmental model. Studies into the early developmental histories of adults with schizophrenia have demonstrated a range of early life anomalies from obstetric complications at birth (Lewis & Murray, 1987; Geddes & Lawrie, 1995), minor physical anomalies such as subtle dysmorphogenesis (the development of abnormal body features) of the craniofacial area (Waddington et al., 1998), and early childhood social and behavioural abnormalities (Watt, 1972). The existence of these anomalies is strongly suggestive of abnormalities in brain function being present from very early in life in people who later develop schizophrenia. However, as they tend to be subtle, non-specific, and have a high frequency in the general population they are weak predictors of schizophrenia (Rapoport et al., 2005). The combination of evidence from these studies and post-mortem studies (which are also suggestive of a neurodevelopmental disturbance) has led to the neurodevelopmental hypothesis of schizophrenia (Weinberger, 1987). One version of the model (early hit) postulates that schizophrenia results from a brain lesion that occurred early in life which affects normal brain development leading to the occurrence of schizophrenia in adolescence or early adulthood (Weinberger, 1987). An alternative version of the developmental model (late hit) suggests that subtle abnormalities of maturational processes that occur during adolescence and early adult life, such as myelination and/or activity-dependent refinement of connections (particularly between limbic and prefrontal cortices) increases the risk of schizophrenia (Egan & Weinberger, 1997; Weinberger & Marenco, 2003). Evidence of a latency period between an early life lesion lying dormant until later brain maturation calls into operation the damaged area exists in epilepsy and dyskinesias (Lewis & Murray, 1987).

Research into genetic factors in schizophrenia has found in family, twin and adoption studies, a long-established familial link in schizophrenia (Gottesman et al., 1987). However, the pattern of inheritance is complex and irregular and many studies have failed to find linkage (Egan & Weinberger, 1997). Although heritability is often estimated to be in the region of 80 per cent, concordance in monozygotic (identical) twins is typically 50 per cent, highlighting the influence of environmental factors (Owen et al., 2005). The polygenic, or multifactorial, model postulates that many genes, each of small effect, combine additively with environmental effects to the aetiology of psychosis (Fowles, 1992). The interaction of many small genetic factors with environmental influences mean that it is highly unlikely that anyone will ever state that they have discovered *the* gene for psychosis or schizophrenia.

Social and environmental influences on psychosis

A multiplicity of environmental factors have been associated with the aetiology of schizophrenia. Some, such as pregnancy and obstetric complications at birth, have been already been discussed, however, there are numerous other environmental factors to consider. Reviews of other reported birth-related factors possibly implicated in the aetiology of schizophrenia included prenatal exposure to rubella, prenatal malnutrition, being born between January to March, being born in urban areas as opposed to rural areas, and elevated rates of diabetes mellitus in the mothers of schizophrenic patients (McDonald & Murray, 2000; Lawrie & Johnstone, 2004). Various other social and environmental factors have also been identified.

That psychoses are socially reactive conditions became an accepted view within psychiatry in the second half of the twentieth century (Bebbington & Kuipers, 2003). The stress-vulnerability model proposed an interaction between individual vulnerability factors such as schizotypal personality traits, biological factors and environmental stressors such as life events and interpersonal difficulties within families (Nuechterlein et al., 1994). Numerous studies (Brown et al., 1962; Leff & Vaughn, 1980; Vaughn et al., 1984) have demonstrated that high expressed emotions (EE) in families, especially those displaying critical comments, hostility and emotional over-involvement may be implicated in the onset of psychosis and increase the risk of psychotic relapse for people with schizophrenia. A review of recent outcome studies has confirmed that the identification of high EE in relatives and close carers with whom people with schizophrenia had a high degree of contact was predictive of subsequent psychotic relapse, conversely implying that social withdrawal acted as a protective factor (Bebbington & Kuipers, 2003). This is interesting because one of the aims of mental health workers seeking to help people with psychotic illnesses is to reduce the amount of social isolation that the individual may be experiencing. Migration is also a risk factor and the risks seem especially high in the offspring of migrants (McDonald & Murray, 2000).

A growing body of evidence has focused on the influence of traumatic early life experiences and the later development of psychosis (Read et al., 2005; Schäfer & Fisher, 2011; Read et al., 2014). Though it has been widely accepted that childhood adversity has a causal role in many adult mental health problems such as depression, anxiety disorders, eating disorders and personality disorders among others (Read et al., 2014), acceptance that it also has a causal role in adult psychosis has been much slower to achieve. The last decade has seen a rapidly expanding body of research into this area (Schäfer & Fisher, 2011). This has led to the continued development of the traumagenic neurodevelopmental model of psychosis. This model seeks to integrate both psychological and biological explanations of psychosis. Psychological processes, such as negative self-appraisal and dissociation, interact with biological processes, such as over reactivity to stress in some brain regions and some structural changes to brain regions including the frontal lobes and the hippocampus (Read et al., 2014), and all of these factors have been implicated in causing psychotic symptoms.

This model has clear implications for practice; first, if a significant number of mental health conditions including psychosis have their origin in childhood adversity, then prevention programmes aimed at targeting social problems such as childhood poverty and early support for vulnerable children and their families may have a positive effect on later development of potential mental health difficulties. Second, it has been suggested (ibid.) that clinicians should routinely ask people if they have experienced childhood adversity. Third, psychological therapies that are aimed at addressing the social causes of their difficulties should be offered to people (ibid.). There now exists evidence (Kumari et al., 2011) that CBT for psychosis can actually attenuate brain responses to threatening stimuli, in other words, the therapy reduced the responses of some parts of the brain to threatening images, indicating that some of the changes caused by adverse experiences can be reversed by therapy.

Research studies into the role of life events have identified the influence that adverse, intrusive, and even exciting life events can have in provoking psychotic relapses. However, the precise nature of the role that life events have in precipitating relapse has produced ambiguous (Bebbington et al., 1993) and inconclusive (Malla et al., 1990) results that are at least partially attributable to methodological differences found in the literature (Fallon, 2008). The question as to whether life events that occur immediately prior to a psychotic episode trigger a relapse or whether the cumulative effect of events over periods as long as a year cause psychotic breakdowns has yet not been answered definitively.

Historical conceptions of psychotic symptoms

As described above, the collection of symptoms that became known as schizophrenia only coalesced as such in the late nineteenth century. Before that people with psychotic symptoms more often attracted the catch-all labels of 'mad' or 'insane'. However, factors such as social status and the ability to function despite one's symptoms could protect some individuals from the negative attitudes of their peers. An early example of this is the Greek philosopher, Socrates. The life and work of Socrates are known mainly to us by the writings of his students Plato and Xenophon, both of whom wrote about a 'voice' that Socrates heard and they noted that he allowed himself to be guided by it. Socrates sometimes described this 'voice' as his 'daemon'. This signifies that his explanation for the existence of a voice talking to him, that only he could hear and was not due to him overhearing another person, was supernatural in nature. However, as Leudar and Thomas (2001) point out, this view was in accordance with the culture of the time where people believed in gods and daemons. This helps us to understand why Socrates accepted this experience without distress and, having discussed it openly with people, was not considered to be ill in any way. Indeed, some believed Socrates to be gifted to be able to hear such a voice (Leudar, 2001). It is often the case that the meaning that one ascribes to an auditory hallucination affects the degree to which it can interfere with everyday life and for Socrates it wasn't seen to be a distressing phenomenon but a privilege (see Figure 5.1).

As was discussed in Chapter 1, after the rise of Christianity the explanations given for bizarre or erratic behaviour across Europe began to be seen as expressions of religious phenomena such as daemonic possession. The loss of the earlier Greek Galenic rationalist approach led to treatments based on a supernatural world view which sought to explain mental illness in terms of demonic possession. However, the Galenic tradition had survived in Islamic medicine and so Islamic societies perceived mental illnesses as deriving from physical causes (usually imbalances in one or more of the four humours). This meant that, in the Islamic world, hospitals

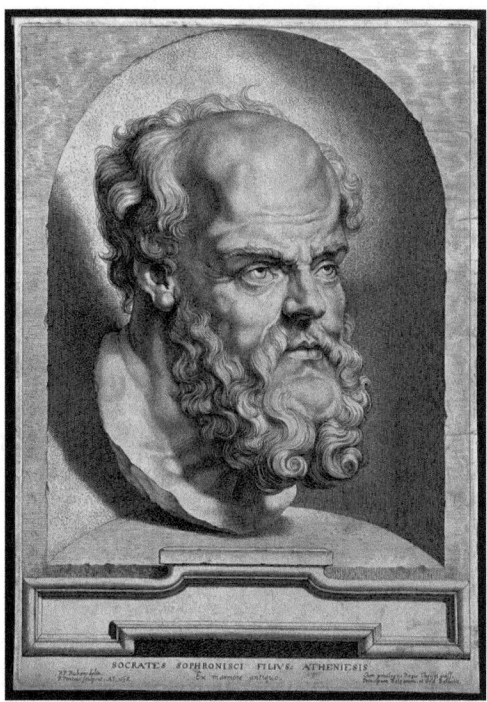

Figure 5.1 Socrates. Line engraving by P. Pontius, 1638, after Sir P. P. Rubens. (Wellcome Collection).

often had wings for the treatment of the mentally ill, with notable examples being in Baghdad and Egypt, from as early as the ninth century (Dols, 1987). These were often spacious and included calming features such as well-tended gardens and fountains. These hospitals adopted a secular approach to the treatment of the mentally ill and surviving medical texts demonstrate a humane and non-moralistic approach (ibid.). Conceptualising madness as having a physical cause led the Islamic physicians to also perceive it as treatable. Drugs used included purgatives, emetics and often the use of opium as a sedative. However, the treatment-regimes were paradoxical in that there are numerous descriptions of people being kept in chains and whipped when they became agitated alongside very enlightened treatments such as baths, massages with oils and musical performances for the patients (ibid.). Though far less influenced by supernatural explanations within the hospital environment, outside the religious supernatural explanations of madness in Islam were strongly felt, especially from the eleventh century on, with the growing influence of Sufism (a term that though contested is usually thought to mean the inner or mystical dimension in Islam) (ibid.). In fact, many Muslims believed in evil spirits (Jinn) and indeed the term used for madness 'junun' literally means 'possession by a Jinn'.

One of the earliest autobiographies by someone that had experienced psychosis is that of an English woman called Margery Kempe, born around 1373. She wrote an autobiography of her life including her mental health problems and the book has been described (Peterson, 1982) as the first fully developed example written in English of an autobiography that describes inner experience. Kempe became ill shortly after the birth of her first child, later stating that she saw and heard flame-tongued devils. She also harmed herself and, at one stage in her illness, needed restraining day and night. She acted strangely, including having many attacks of crying loudly in public, often in response to religious visions she experienced, which indicates that there was a hysterical component to her psychotic illness. She became convinced that it was angels and God himself talking to her and she devoted herself to a life of chastity (though by this time she had given birth to 14 children) and the service of God (Porter, 1989). Though her initial illness seems possibly to be an example of puerperal psychosis, i.e. triggered by the stress of childbirth, Margery continued to experience both auditory and visual hallucinations. Given the religious nature of the times she lived in this was seen by some as evidence of great religious piety and by others as heresy, indeed she was tried for heresy in 1407 but was acquitted. It appears that because her experiences took on a singularly religious character this not only brought her to the attention of the clergy in a way that could endanger her but also meant that she was perceived by others as a religious mystic rather than someone with mental health issues.

A contemporary of Margery Kempe was the French king, Charles VI (1368–1422) also known as 'Charles the mad'. He suffered from numerous episodes of psychosis, including the delusion that he was Saint George. When ill, Charles became fearful and paranoid and was usually confined to his residence. Another delusion that he suffered from has become known as *glass delusion*; this was very common in the Middle Ages. For Charles it took the form of a fear that he would shatter if he bumped into anything too firmly and, to protect himself, he had iron rods sewn into his clothes. Charles has been described as one of the first people to be afflicted with this particular delusion (Pietikainen, 2015) and it may be that it became more common due to an early sufferer being a king. This indicates that, though for some it may have been a delusion (fixed false belief) which is a psychotic symptom, for others it may have been driven more by individual anxieties which then found form in the glass delusion. Pietikainen (ibid.) describes it as an obsession driven by people's sense of vulnerability (life expectancy was short in the Middle Ages), again indicating that the same symptom (a fear of being made of glass and hence very fragile) could be, for some, psychotic in nature but for others could be an expression of their everyday worries about life. Glass delusion persisted for over 200 years and it is mentioned by Burton in his *The Anatomy of Melancholy* in 1621 and in popular culture by figures as varied as Hobbes, Cervantes, Huygens and Descartes. The glass delusion almost disappeared after the advent of the early modern age though there have been a couple of modern examples, one being the Canadian pianist Glenn Gould (1932–1982) who was always fearful of being touched too firmly.

Views of madness have never been static and, even within a particular historical period, various views could coexist with each other so, for example, though the predominant view in Western Europe could for centuries be in the main shaped by religious (predominantly Christian) superstitions, others viewed the mentally ill as 'lunatics', 'melancholic' or 'deranged'. However, as long as the predominant explanation was religious the main cures were also religious not least among them exorcism. In 1677 the German painter Christoph Haizmann experienced seizures while attending church. When the seizures lasted into a second day he was taken to the prefect of Pottenbrunn and confessed that, nine years earlier while depressed after the death of one of his parents, he had entered into a pact with Satan. The devil would help Haizmann with his life and at the end of nine years he would give himself over, body and soul, to the devil. The nine years would be up within a month and Haizmann begged to be sent to a shrine at Mariazell. At Mariazell, Haizmann submitted himself to three days of continuous exorcism and prayer. At midnight of the third day the devil appeared to him in the form of a dragon holding the written pact Haizmann had signed in his own blood. He snatched it from the devil and immediately the seizures stopped. Haizmann stayed for a while at Mariazell and painted nine paintings of his experiences with the devil, which are still in existence.

Unfortunately for Haizmann, after a month the seizures and terrifying visions returned and so, nine months later, he returned to Mariazell asking for a second exorcism. This second exorcism was apparently successful and he remained at the convent until his death in 1700. Porter (1989) has pointed out that within Haizmann's diary of his experiences and other contemporaneous accounts there is no mention of the word 'insanity' as it appears that at that time in Austria such religious experiences were not thought of as necessarily a sign of mental illness. However, Porter also states that while this was true for Haizmann, it was not the case for an English contemporary of his, George Trosse. Trosse (1631–1713) also wrote an account of his life that gives us an insight into the lived experiences of a person who experienced psychosis centuries ago. In Trosse's account he describes being a vain young man partial to alcohol who, after one heavy drinking session, saw a spirit and then heard a voice talking to him which he initially concluded was the voice of God but later due to its demands, he realized was the devil. Trosse goes on to describe numerus hallucinations and delusions where including one of when he was taken to see a physician in Glastonbury he was given a glass of water to drink out of and thought it turned black and that it was a great black fly or beetle which was actually the devil and, by drinking it, he allowed himself to be possessed by the devil. Trosse was confined in the asylum there and, as the doctor's wife soothed and prayed with him, gradually calmed and the delusions subsided (ibid.). However, after returning home he returned to his old licentious ways and became delusional again. In all, it took three stays at Glastonbury for Trosse to become well. The main treatment apart from confinement appears to have been the ministrations of Mrs Gollop, the doctor's wife, which was successful since he went on to study at Oxford and become a well-known nonconformist minister. What is interesting is that, though Trosse's delusions were religious in character, the response was not wholly religious – though he was prayed with and this was done in the confines of a madhouse not a convent, as was the case for Haizmann (see Figure 5.2).

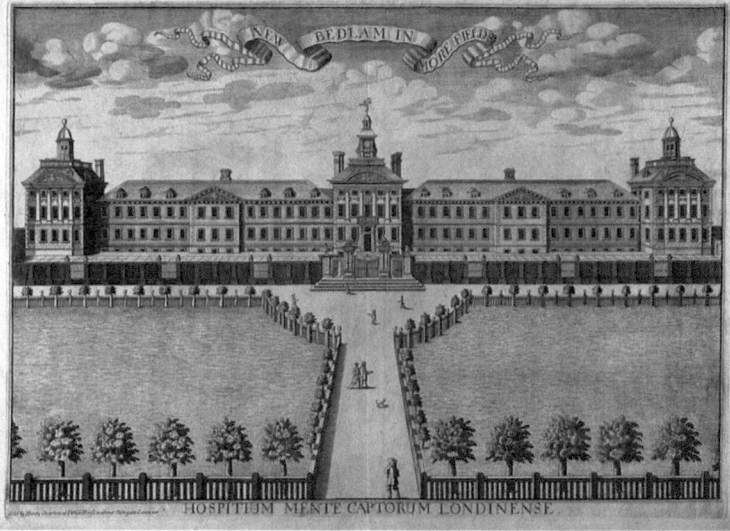

Figure 5.2 The hospital of Bethlem [Bedlam] at Moorfields: The entrance facade. Engraving by A. Soly. (Wellcome Collection).

The coming of the enlightenment and the intellectual, scientific and philosophical changes in thought it brought led to significant changes in European societies, including an undermining of the demonological view of the world that was prevalent up until that point. One noticeable example was the decline in the trials and executions of women for witchcraft. The last execution for witchcraft took place in England in 1684. Another was a move to describe the world in different, less religious/more secular ways, a host of philosophers (often with differing views) including Descartes, Hobbes and Locke all saw humans as rational beings and the world a place that could be explained by rational, not supernatural, theories. At the same time as philosophers brought changes in ways of looking at the world, scientists and medical men, such as Thomas Willis, discovered new ways of looking at the human body that undermined the old humoral view. The discovery of the nervous system led to new theories of how physical and mental disorders were interconnected. Just as the religious treatments of prayer and exorcism diminished so did the Galenic ones of emetics, bloodletting and the like. However, as Porter (2004) has pointed out, it would be an oversimplification to state that the scientific and philosophical changes happening in Europe had any immediate effect on the treatment of people for either physical or mental illnesses. These changes occurred gradually and unevenly across European countries throughout the seventeenth, and well into the eighteenth, centuries.

The development of the asylum

These societal changes also influenced exactly where people with mental health problems were cared for. On the whole, throughout Europe in the Middle Ages, people with mental health difficulties were cared for privately at home as there were few institutions to care for them. This also meant that they were also very visible to the general public if they did not have relatives to care for them, as they would often be out in public. There were some small private 'madhouses' and monasteries that took in people, however, in England, Wales and Ireland due to the dissolution of the monasteries during the Reformation there were far fewer of these establishments.

England did create Europe's first psychiatric hospital, Bethlehem Hospital; which was founded in 1247, and became exclusively for people with mental illnesses in the late fourteenth or early fifteenth centuries (the exact date is now disputed). Despite its infamy and being responsible for the term 'bedlam' as a corruption of Bethlam (which itself was a corruption of the word Bethlehem), for several centuries it housed a very small number of patients, for example in 1598 a committee of inspection found that it only had 20 'inmates' (Arnold, 2009). This is important because the French philosopher Michel Foucault had argued that the period from roughly 1660 to 1800 during the Enlightenment was the era of the 'great confinement' when bourgeois society wanted to remove the workless, feckless and mentally ill from view and have greater control over them by locking them all up together.

Though there are many insights in Foucault's work pertaining to societal views of deviance and mental illness, and the attempts of European states to silence deviants by removing them from society, there are problems with his theory. For example, the increase in number of people incarcerated in England remained very small throughout this period. The poor were helped by the policy not of incarceration but of outdoor relief until the Poor Law Amendment Act of 1834, which instituted the era of the workhouse. Porter (2004) pointed out that even in France, where Foucault begins his analysis, the actual number of people confined during Foucault's period of study remained low, though it was rising. Across the rest of Europe— especially peasant Europe—including Ireland, Spain, Portugal and Russia, there was no growth in custodial institutions and the Church remained an important source of support for the ill and the destitute. Furthermore, not all the 'inmates' in private asylums were the poor mentally ill, as these institutions survived as private businesses by having wealthy paying customers. Therefore, though there was a growth in the number of institutions for people deemed to be 'mad' or lacking reason during the period Foucault spoke about, for the most part these were small private undertakings with few inmates and it wasn't until during the nineteenth century that Europe saw the advent of the large-scale asylum.

There were also other changes occurring in the late eighteenth century in response to this modest growth in asylums and to broader political factors, which included some degree of state control over asylums and some attempts to reform their worse practices. Therefore, in England, Parliament passed legislation requiring a physician, surgeon or apothecary to fill out a medical certificate before confining non-pauper patients (this didn't apply to paupers who could still be confined as others in society saw fit). The late eighteenth century was also the period of the American War of Independence and the French Revolution, both of which encouraged radical ideas across Europe. In France, three years after the revolution in 1792 Pinel, the new director of the Bicêtre Hospital, looked at conditions on the seventh ward where 200 mentally ill men were kept. He introduced humane forms of treatment and ended practices such as bleeding and purging. This encouraged the later removal of chains from the patients, something he repeated at his next post at the Hospice de la Salpêtrière (Porter, 1989). At the same time, in England the Quaker William Tuke, horrified by the conditions that mentally ill people were kept in, set up his own asylum, the York Retreat, which opened in 1796. Again, older practices such as bleeding were not allowed and there were no chains. Treatments included warm baths, exercise and taking up hobbies. These changes occurred gradually and unevenly; a government commission into Bethlehem Hospital reported to the House of Commons in 1815 that one of the female patients had been chained up for 8 years and that a male patient named William Norris had been chained for 14 years (Arnold, 2009). Even as late as 1837, another report into conditions at Bethlehem found that some patients were still chained (see Figure 5.3).

One inhabitant of an early nineteenth century English madhouse that highlights both the brutal treatment meted out at some asylums and the better more enlightened care from others is John Perceval (1803–1876). Perceval was the son of Prime Minister Spencer Perceval who has the dubious honour of being the only British prime minister to be assassinated in office (in 1812 when John was nine). As an aside, the man who shot Spencer Perceval, John Bellingham, was thought to be mentally ill but, as his trial started only four days after the murder, he pleaded not guilty stating he had not been given time to mount a defence. However, His lawyers thought him mentally unwell and tried to mount an insanity defence, though the court

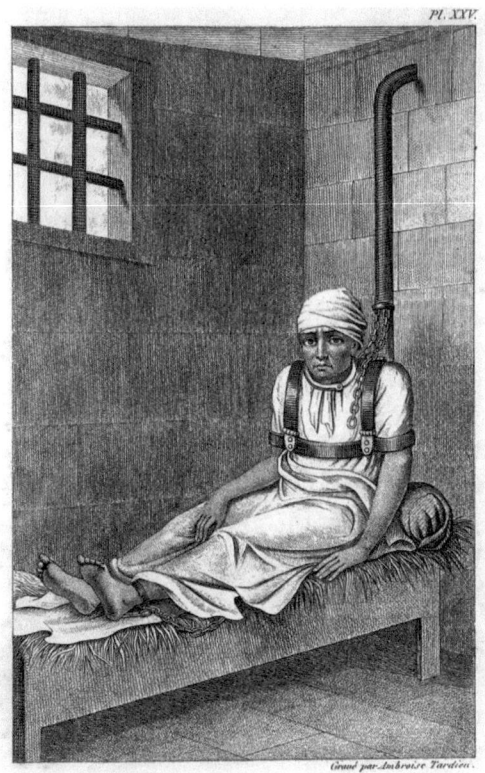

Figure 5.3 William Norris, shackled on his bed at Bedlam. (Wellcome Collection).

rejected—it partly because Bellingham himself declared he was not insane. In what is now thought to be a serious miscarriage of justice Bellingham was found guilty and hung on the 18 May 1812, just 1 week after he shot Perceval. A number of years later, in 1831 when John was 27, his mental health deteriorated after two significant events. First, always a religious man, he had visited a religious sect in Scotland that spoke in tongues and submitted to their spontaneous impulses, something he apparently took to enthusiastically. Second, after this he visited Dublin in Ireland and, after contracting a sexually transmitted disease from a prostitute, he was treated with mercury, it is thought that the combination of these two events led to John losing contact with reality.

During his illness Perceval saw visions and heard voices. His brother brought him back to England and his family paid for him to be 'cared' for in private asylums. He later wrote two volumes of recollections of his experiences in the asylums. These detail the inhumane ways in which he was treated and, from the investigations into Bethlehem described above, it appears that throughout England there were as many cruel regimes as there were enlightened ones. Perceval's reason for publishing his memoires was to draw attention to the treatment of the mentally ill and to argue for reform of legislation regarding the management of the asylums and the treatment of their charges. He describes enforced cold baths, beatings, restraints and forced medical treatments. Peterson (1982) has pointed out that the two volumes also give us a rare insight into Perceval's experiences of psychosis and how he believes such people should be treated by those around them. Perceval recounted uncaring, even humiliating, treatment at the hands of those paid to care for him. After around a year at one asylum he was moved to another, Ticehurst House, where he received better care – in all he spent around three years in asylums. In 1845, Perceval joined the Alleged Lunatics' Friend Society to continue campaigning for patients' rights. In 1859 he gave evidence to a parliamentary select committee, unfortunately it did not result in any new reforming legislation and it appears the activity of the Society petered out soon afterwards. Perceval deserves to be remembered as an early advocate for patient's rights and for mental health reform.

Asylums in America could be just as inhumane. The reporter Elizabeth Cochran, in one of the first pieces of undercover reporting, spent ten days in the Women's Lunatic Asylum on Blackwell's Island near Manhattan in 1887 – she described the rotten food, rough treatment from staff and the rat infestation that made the place intolerable. Her book *Ten Days in a Mad-House* (written under her pen name of Nellie Bly) caused a sensation and a subsequent Grand Jury investigation led to changes in the asylum system and an increase in the budget of the department that funded asylums.

The asylum wasn't only a European and North American institution. Due to the colonial expansion of European countries, asylums were opened across the globe. Keller (2001) makes the point that under colonial rule, where the ruling state is in a state of tension with the local population, psychiatric knowledge when used to incarcerate local people has a powerful and complex position within society. The history of colonial psychiatry, like the history of much of colonialism, highlights the inherent racism used to justify colonial rule. In India the process of development followed the European model; initially the asylums were small private concerns that became bigger and came under state ownership from the 1850s onwards as the British administrative presence increased. The larger asylums in cities such as Calcutta and Mumbai catered mainly to European patients. Unlike in Britain where work for inmates was seen as constructive, in India it was seen as injurious to European patients, whereas Indian patients were forced into intensive labour (ibid.). Unlike Britain, where mechanical restraints had largely disappeared they continued to be used by European psychiatrists in India much later into the nineteenth century where the task of restraining European patients fell to orderlies and nurses, all of whom were Indian.

A different picture emerged in Africa where the colonial presence did not immediately lead to the growth of asylums. There was a delay in their development, with British and French mental health institutions developing in the twentieth century long after the arrival of the colonialists. The reasons given (ibid.) are that health care was focused on the more dangerous tropical diseases prevalent in sub-Saharan Africa and that, unlike India where the British East India Company provided financing for hospitals, there was no equivalent large company operating in Africa. Geography also had a part to play, especially with France being much closer to North Africa than Britain was to India, making it easier to transport violent and or disturbed European and indigenous patients to asylums in southern France.

The nineteenth century was the era of the growth of the asylums. An era where reforms removed the strait jackets and shackles across Europe. It was also the time of the development of the discipline of psychiatry. Porter (1989) has estimated that in 1800 around 5,000 people were incarcerated in asylums in Britain and that this rocketed to 100,000 by 1900. Though the use of moral rather than physical force was progressive, it is also true that the development of large public-run asylums warehoused many individuals and became more overcrowded and impersonal than the old private asylums had been. Though mechanical restraints became less common all sorts of medicinal ones were still used. Opium was commonly used to sedate agitated patients, for example. This was before the development of specific antipsychotic medication. Consider, for example, the German Judge Daniel Schreber who was hospitalised in Leipzig in 1894 experiencing multiple delusions and hallucinations. He made so much noise shouting out at night that the local population complained to the hospital authorities who then encouraged him to sleep in a padded cell until his night time outbursts eventually lessened— over two years later!

At the turn of the twentieth century, as asylums around the globe but especially in Europe, the USA and colonial Asia and Africa continued to expand, there were still accounts of very poor treatment written by former inmates. One such account was by Clifford Beers (1876–1943) who spent two years in various private and public asylums. Beers had been working on Wall Street when he became ill. His older brother had suffered from seizures and a brain tumour, eventually dying, and Beers worried that this would happen to him. As is sometimes the case, people who fear the worst (death usually) find the wait for its arrival more intolerable than the feared thing itself and Beers decided that he should kill himself. In 1900 he jumped from the fourth floor of his family home and broke some bones in his feet. At this point it appears he was experiencing anxiety and probably depression, however, after he was hospitalised he continued to ruminate and began to think that he was not in hospital but in prison (they had put bars on his windows to prevent him jumping again). He became psychotic and among his delusions he believed his family had been replaced by doubles (this particular delusion is known as 'Capgras delusion' after the French psychiatrist Joseph Capgras who was the first to describe it), that his food was poisoned and that the staff were undercover police. He remained largely mute throughout the two-year period. He later wrote about it in a book that became a best seller, *A Mind that Found Itself* (Peterson, 1982). In it he recounts the brutal treatment from staff including physical violence, forced feeding and the use of straitjackets that he endured and saw other inmates experience. Like Perceval 70 years earlier, Beers became well known for his account of his illness and (mis)treatment. Also like Perceval, he set up an organisation based on his experiences – his National Committee for Mental Hygiene – though it didn't aim to improve conditions for those with mental health issues, it was more aimed at encouraging self-help and education aimed at maintaining good mental health. The Mental Hygiene Movement became the first large-scale educative movement for better mental health, it raised millions of dollars and made Beers very well known. Sadly, he ended his days back in an asylum in 1943 after further relapses into psychosis.

Treatments of psychosis

Throughout the first half of the twentieth century psychiatrists tried all sorts of treatments to quell the furious minds of their patients with schizophrenia. At the core of these treatments was the view of psychiatrists throughout much of Europe, though especially in France, Britain and in the USA, that schizophrenia was essentially a physical illness of the brain. One of the earliest proponents of this view was the French psychiatrist Morel, who argued in an influential work in 1857 that the mentally ill belonged to those classes in society that were biologically and morally inferior to the rest of society (Scull, 2015). It thus followed that treatments should be physical in nature rather than psychological. Germany was an exception to this approach as German research focused at a cellular level seeking to discover the causes of mental illnesses in the nerves and especially in the brain, an example being the studies of Alzheimer into the plaques and tangles in the brain that cause a specific type of dementia (ibid.). The era from the late nineteenth and into the twentieth century was also the era of psychoanalysis but Freud, and other psychologists interested in people with psychosis (Freud studied and theorised on the case of Daniel Schreber extensively for example), realised that people so out of contact with reality were not suitable cases for talking therapies and concentrated their therapeutic endeavours on people with 'neurotic' (essentially anxiety and depression) disorders.

A very common treatment given to patients in this era was insulin coma therapy (ICT) and a particularly famous recipient of it was the ballet dancer Nijinsky (1889 to 1950). Nijinsky is regarded as one of the world's finest-ever ballet dancers. After a breakdown in relationships with his ballet company, a difficult marriage, interruptions to his dancing due to the First World War and the stress of both being principle dancer and tour manager, Nijinsky suffered some kind of breakdown while on tour in Uruguay. As he became more erratic and suspicious, his wife took him to see Bleuler himself who, after a short interview, diagnosed Nijinsky as schizophrenic. After this, he spent most of the rest of his life in and out of institutions. He was given insulin coma therapy in 1938 – in this treatment doses of insulin were given to a person until they reached a dose that induced a coma. Seizures sometimes occurred before or during the coma; which was terminated after about an hour by giving the person glucose, either intravenously or by nasogastric tube. Interestingly, similar to electroconvulsive therapy (ECT) another of the so called 'shock therapies' for reasons that remain largely unknown, such seizures can have a positive effect on mental health conditions and it was noted that Nijinsky did briefly improve after a course of them. Unfortunately, on the whole he remained very ill for the rest of his life. In general, ICT was given due to a lack of alternatives and was often given to patients thought to have a good prognosis, therefore they may have been likely to improve anyway. Though it became a standard treatment in Britain and the US in the 1930s and 1940s, after the discovery of antipsychotic drugs its use declined rapidly. It also often gave rise to very serious side effects such as obesity, brain damage and in some cases death.

As more and more people accumulated in asylums throughout the nineteenth and into the twentieth century in large parts of the world, it became clear that few treatments were genuinely effective in treating the more serious mental illnesses such as mania and psychosis (Shorter, 1997). This therapeutic pessimism and the discovery of genuine treatments, such as insulin for diabetes, also drove the search for 'cures' to psychotic illnesses. Insulin coma therapy was one such example but was not the only one. Others included malarial therapy; which was a treatment for General Paralysis of the Insane (GPI), a condition caused by contracting syphilis. This involved injecting blood infected with malaria into an individual to cause a fever that would destroy the parasite and arrest the decline into madness then death that accompanied GPI. Results seemed to indicate some success though it was a dangerous approach as not all those treated responded well to the quinine used to cure the malaria. It was then tried on many psychiatric conditions, including schizophrenia, with less impressive results. However, the discoverer and main proponent of malarial therapy, Julius Wagner-Jauregg, became the first psychiatrist to win the Nobel Prize for Medicine in 1927.

Another 'treatment' being pioneered in the first half of the twentieth century led to its founder becoming the second winner of a Nobel Prize for Psychiatry. The recipient was the Portuguese neurologist Egas Moniz (in 1949). Moniz experimented on 20 patients diagnosed with schizophrenia to see if destroying tissue in the frontal lobes of their brains improved their psychotic symptoms. He swiftly published a paper describing improvement in 14 of the patients. Given the lack of follow up and lack of statistical rigour (ibid.), these claims should be treated extremely cautiously. However, despite this, the procedure was taken up enthusiastically especially in the USA where it was renamed as *lobotomy*. One of the main proponents of it, Walter Freeman, refined the procedure to such an extent that he was able to perform many operations in a day. This was the *transorbital lobotomy* whereby an ice pick was hammered just above the eye ball into the brain and then moved in a sweeping motion in order to sever brain tissue. In the US between 1940 and 1944, 684 lobotomies were carried out and, by its peak year of 1949, 5,074 were carried out (ibid.). One unfortunate recipient of a lobotomy was Rose Williams (1909–1996), the older sister of the playwright Tennessee Williams. Her life inspired several of her brother's characters including Laura in *The Glass Menagerie*. As she entered her twenties her behaviour became more erratic and she was eventually placed in the state hospital in Farmington. After numerous treatments, including insulin shock therapy, failed to help she was given a bilateral prefrontal lobotomy in 1943. Unfortunately, despite early hopes that she had improved, she subsequently deteriorated further after the surgery and spent the rest of her life in psychiatric institutions. Though Moniz won the Nobel Prize for his role in the development of lobotomies, there were always many that worked in mental health who were uncomfortable about it and its use died out quickly after the advent of the age of antipsychotics.

As has been discussed earlier, doctors and others treating the mentally ill have for centuries tried to find drugs that could help their patients. Various potions were used as purgatives (laxatives) and others, such as opium and chloral hydrate, also had extensive histories as agents used to calm and sedate disturbed people. These, and other drugs, gave nothing more than temporary relief to the individual and were not thought of as cures. The discovery of medication that was effective in treating psychotic symptoms such as auditory hallucinations was one of the most significant developments in treating psychosis in the twentieth century. As with many drug discoveries, the finding that a certain type of drug (a phenothiazine) was an effective antipsychotic occurred by accident. The first two (promethazine and chlorpromazine) were initially used as antihistamines and then, subsequently, to increase the effects of anaesthetics. This led to the discovery by a French military surgeon, Henri Laborit, in 1952 that they had significant effects on the central nervous system and he and a colleague, Pierre Huguenard, persuaded psychiatrists at two hospitals in Paris to try chlorpromazine on their patients. The effects on patients who had previously been agitated and experiencing severe psychotic symptoms were transformative, as many became calmer and their psychotic symptoms reduced greatly and, in some cases, disappeared totally. No other treatment had ever had such an effect.

Psychiatrists in France produced numerous papers reporting on the effects of chlorpromazine throughout the first half of 1952. By November 1952 chlorpromazine, under its trade name Largactil, became available on prescription. By 1955, its use had spread around the world (Ban, 2007). Such positive results led scientists to search for more and more antipsychotic compounds, which resulted in many new drugs coming onto the market. One thing that is important to note is that for a number of years no one knew what the mechanism of action was by which chlorpromazine was able reduce psychotic symptoms. That it does work can be seen from the experiences of people such as Mark Vonnegut (1947–), the son of writer Kurt Vonnegut, who has written about his psychotic breakdown in 1971, which he attributed to stress and the use of psychedelic drugs. After his friends in the commune in which he was living attempted to help him without medical interventions, without success, he was taken to a hospital in Vancouver. He was experiencing voices, visions and paranoia and was treated with Thorazine (a trade name for chlorpromazine) and recovered. However, after discharge he discontinued his medication and relapsed necessitating a readmission to hospital where the medication was reintroduced, helping him to recover again (Peterson, 1982).

Within two years of the introduction of antipsychotics it became clear that they were often accompanied by a range of side effects that could have a distressing, and sometimes debilitating, effect on the user. Despite demonstrated clinical effectiveness in reducing psychotic symptoms, the long-term use of antipsychotics is clearly associated with adverse neurological effects, especially the induction of several movement disorders – acute extrapyramidal side effects (EPSE) and tardive dyskinesia (TD) (Barnes, 1992). EPSE is most associated with drug-induced parkinsonism and akathisia. Drug-induced parkinsonism closely resembles idiopathic Parkinson's disease, especially the presence of tremor, rigidity and bradykinesia (abnormally slow voluntary movements), (ibid.). Akathisia is a subjective feeling of inner restlessness, often accompanied by objective signs such as pacing and an inability to keep the legs still (ibid.). Other side effects of the first antipsychotics included sedation and slowed thinking. The Nobel Prize winning mathematician John Nash stopped taking antipsychotic medication in 1970 despite the dream-like delusional hypotheses he described in the autobiographical essay he submitted to the Nobel Committee because he believed they blunted his intellect.

Modern antipsychotics are usually described as 'atypical' because they don't cause (or cause to a lesser degree) the movement disorders that the older drugs caused. However, they can still cause considerable side effects such as weight gain and associated metabolic conditions such as hyperlipidaemia and type 2 diabetes. It is always vital that when people are commenced on such medication that the possible side effects are explained to them. For example, for those drugs that stimulate appetite it is vital that this potential is explained so that people can try to control their portion size when they begin taking the medication. It is also routine practice in the UK to take baseline measures such as weight and a range of blood tests to monitor any changes that occur after the medication has commenced.

Though antipsychotic medication works for many people the effects are variable. Some people respond very well to antipsychotic medication, some respond partially and some people receive no benefit at all from them. There is a large degree of trial and error with these drugs as one can never be sure which particular antipsychotic will be beneficial to any one person at which dose and to what degree. This means that, despite the clinical benefits that they have brought, there remains considerable criticism of them. It has been argued (Bentall & Morrison, 2002) that given these potential negative effects, antipsychotics should not be used as a preventative measure in high-risk populations such as young people exhibiting brief psychotic symptoms, or with a strong family history of psychosis.

Other drugs, especially illicit hallucinogenic drugs, mimic some of the symptoms of psychosis. For some people with a vulnerability to develop a psychotic illness such drugs can trigger an episode of illness. There are numerous examples of people who have had their mental health damaged by using hallucinogens; such as Syd Barrett the original Pink Floyd guitarist, Brian Wilson from the Beach Boys and Pete Green the guitarist from Fleetwood Mac. Green was taking large amounts of LSD and this affected his behaviour. He became erratic and obsessed with not wanting to make money. He left Fleetwood Mac in 1970 and has spent time in psychiatric hospitals. From the late seventies onwards he gradually moved back into playing music in various bands. He has stated that he still experiences auditory hallucinations despite taking various medication over the years.

Given the history of coercive treatment of people with psychosis, ignoring the opinions of people due to a perception of them as 'mad' and therefore out of contact with reality in every instance, invasive procedures and variable response rates to medication that often causes side effects, it is entirely understandable that there have always been campaigns against the psychiatric establishment. John Perceval's campaigns for better treatment and care in the nineteenth century are a good early example of this. Some, such as the antipsychiatry movement which began in the 1960s, have come from the practitioners themselves whereas others have come from the service user movement or a combination of practitioners and service users. Some have argued (Romme et al., 1992) that rather than always seeking to 'treat' the individual's perception of reality it could be more useful to accept their perception of reality and discuss their subjective experience of hearing voices. In their research Romme et al. (ibid.) identified a variety of coping strategies that people who hear voices use to cope with them, especially distraction techniques such as watching a film, engaging in physical exercise or meditating. It has long been understood that people who are more distressed experience worse psychotic symptoms, including hearing voices. Therefore it follows that, if people can gain some understanding of what their 'voices' mean to them then they may become less fearful of them and therefore less distressed, which may have a positive impact on the intensity and frequency of their experiences.

Marius Romme (born 1934) has been instrumental in setting up the Hearing Voices Network (HVN) which seeks to challenge many of the accepted ideas around hearing voices, such as that they are always a symptom of schizophrenia and that the 'sufferer' must be 'treated' with antipsychotic medication. The HVN conceptualises voice hearing as similar to dreams and they are comfortable with people generating their own explanations for their experiences. They advocate the individual getting as much information as possible to make informed choices about their treatment but stress the importance of talking therapies and state that though medication is useful for some people it should be a matter of choice. Again, one of the best evidenced talking therapies is CBT where the interpretation (beliefs about) of the unusual experience is seen as central to how distressed the person becomes and how they react to their experiences. The person is then encouraged to assess the evidence for their beliefs and try with the help of their therapist to develop alternative explanations for their distressing experiences. Undermining the strength they have in a certain explanation for their experiences can reduce the amount of distress they experience.

One influential person involved in the hearing voices network is Rufus May (born 1968) who has worked as a clinical psychologist in mental health in England for over 20 years. He has also used his own experiences of becoming psychotic at the age of 18 to inform his practice and views on treatments of psychosis. He has written (May

& Svanholmer, 2016) about believing at that time that many people and animals were actually robots and that a gadget had been put in his chest to control him. May took antipsychotic medication for over a year before he decided to wean himself off it. This he found difficult to do but, since then, he has successfully managed his mental health in other ways. He advocates developing support networks so that people do not feel socially isolated; something that can exacerbate auditory hallucinations and paranoid thoughts. He has also found being among people who accept that there is more than one way to experience reality helpful. Within this approach is an inherent criticism of statutory mental health services that see their view of reality as 'objective' and that of the person with psychosis as 'subjective' and therefore seek to 'treat' rather than engage with the person's alternate view of reality. Statutory services are supportive of the aims of the recovery movement. This movement grew out of grass-roots service-user initiatives in the 1980s and has spread over large parts of the world. The essence of its philosophy is that services should adopt a sense of hope and optimism towards service users. Furthermore, recovery doesn't necessarily mean recovery from a condition as is the case in a medical model but recovery within the context of one's condition. For example, for some people this may well be working full-time whereas for others it could be attending a drop-in or support group to reduce their social isolation.

One of the many positive impacts of the HVN is that it has now become much less stigmatising for public figures to talk about their experiences of hearing voices. For example, Jon Ronson, the investigative journalist, has spoken about how he heard voices in his head as a child when he went to bed and Graham Linehan, the writer and director, has also spoken about his experiences of hearing voices. What is interesting is that this increase in people who are highly successful in their chosen fields talking about their experiences of hearing voices or other psychotic experiences reinforces the view that such experiences are far more common than just confined to those people who receive the diagnosis 'schizophrenia'. Psychosis is often understandable in terms of the individual's life experiences. It is a range of experiences that are also treatable with a range of therapeutic interventions that make a recovery-orientated approach meaningful.

6

Bipolar Disorder

The World Health Organization estimates that bipolar disorder affects approximately 60 million people worldwide (WHO, 2018a). It is the fourth most common mental disorder behind depression, anxiety and schizophrenia. Bipolar disorder has a high rate of reoccurrence, however, unlike schizophrenia the degree of chronicity is much lower (Angst & Sellaro, 2000). Therefore, more people are likely to recover a degree of functionality between episodes, though length of illness and number of manic episodes has been shown to affect social functioning negatively (Lam et al., 1999). Unfortunately, due to the impact of episodes of illness there is a lifetime prevalence of suicide attempts of up to 30 per cent (Bauer & Pfennig, 2005) which is higher than for any other psychiatric disorder.

Most studies have found no difference in the rates of bipolar disorder between men and women and it appears to affect between 1 and 1.5 per cent of the adult population (Lam et al., 1999). Bipolar disorder usually occurs in adolescence or young adult years (Bauer & Pfennig, 2005) and an earlier age of onset is associated with poorer outcomes and more episodes of illness. The disorder seems to be greater in ethnic minority communities (Lloyd et al., 2005) especially where the ethnic minority is a small proportion of the local population. People with bipolar disorder also often have comorbid conditions such as anxiety disorders, attention deficit hyperactivity disorder (ADHD), alcohol and drug dependence (Miklowitz & Johnson, 2006). The social costs of bipolar disorder are significant as many people experience periodic reoccurrences of symptoms which affect their ability to sustain careers and relationships.

Given that one pole of bipolar disorder is depression it is not uncommon for people who initially present with a depressive episode to be diagnosed as depressed and only be reclassified as bipolar when they subsequently present with a hypomanic or manic episode. Therefore, it has been argued that there can be delays of between 5 and 10 years between the first episode of illness and receiving treatment (Bauer & Pfennig, 2005) and that bipolar disorder is a considerably underdiagnosed condition (Angst et al., 2010).

Bipolar disorder is a disorder where the individual has two or more episodes of significantly disturbed mood (WHO, 2018c). Some of these episodes will be of an elevated mood (mania or hypomania, which is milder in character) including symptoms such as increased energy, overactive behaviour, talking rapidly (pressure of speech), decreased need for sleep and distractibility. They also often exhibit grandiose ideas such as a belief that they possess vast sums of money and this can lead to significant problems if they spend money they don't actually possess.

Sometimes when people experience an elevated mood, what is commonly described as a 'manic' phase they may also experience psychotic symptoms. This demonstrates both how mental health conditions can overlap and how difficult it can be to accurately diagnose the person presenting in front of you. Other episodes of illness may be a feeling of low mood which itself can be of varying severity from mild depression to being severely depressed. Obviously, if a person first presents with a depressive episode then they will most likely be considered suffering from depression. It is only over time when they subsequently have an episode of elevated (hypomanic or manic) mood that it will become clear that they have bipolar disorder. The same is true if they initially present with a hypomanic episode (persistent mild elevation of mood) or manic episode as these can sometimes happen to people who have been under significant stress and can be a 'one-off' event and clinicians are, therefore, cautious of diagnosing bipolar disorder from one presentation. However, over time if they then have a depressive episode and further periods of elevated mood, bipolar disorder would be diagnosed. To be diagnosed as a manic episode it has to last at least seven days or require hospitalisation (ibid.).

Of all the categories of mental distress 'bipolar disorder' is the one that seems to have attracted the most attention in the media in recent years. This is because it has positive as well as negative connotations attached to it. It has long been associated with both creativity and genius and so has a positive counterbalance to the usual stigma that major mental health issues attract. The term *bipolar* is itself a relatively recent development in this particular condition, for many years it was described as 'manic depression'. *Mania* was up until the mid-nineteenth century the catch-all term for those people who presented as 'mad', 'deranged', 'disturbed' or other such terms, and would therefore have included people who today would be described as having conditions including delirium, schizophrenia, other psychoses and bipolar disorder. Therefore for centuries 'mania' included vast numbers of mentally ill people. Those people who we would now describe as having affective, i.e. mood, disorders such as depression, anxiety etc. would have attracted a diagnosis of melancholia.

Development of the concept of bipolar disorder

One of the earliest descriptions of bipolar disorder was made by the Greek physician Aretaeus of Cappadocia, he wrote clinical descriptions of a number of medical and mental disorders. He described how euphoria can follow melancholy and suggested that the two may be linked which, considering he was writing around 150 AD, was a remarkable insight. He was a remarkable physician who was also credited with describing and giving the name to diabetes and giving the first clinical description of celiac disease. Unfortunately, both he and his works were forgotten for centuries and only rediscovered and published in the sixteenth century (Tekiner, 2015).

Attempts to classify mental illnesses into more distinct categories than mania and melancholia flourished in the nineteenth century. In the mid- to late-nineteenth century the most common perception of mania was that it was a chronic condition that began as chronic over excitement and gradually developed into mental degeneration, poor memory and other symptoms of dementia. Some thought that up to half the cases would make a full recovery

(Hare, 1981). However, the general perception was that both mania and melancholia led, in many cases, to a chronic dementia state that needed caring for in asylums. One English textbook of the time (Bucknill & Tuke, 1858) was typical in its view of what the causes of mania were; these included moral causes such as anxiety, disappointed affections, jealousy, excessive joy from prosperity, any intense mental emotion or strain on the intellectual powers, fright, ambition, ungratified and wounded vanity or self-esteem. Among physical causes were listed; hereditary predisposition, intemperance, injuries of the head, fever, disappearance of a cutaneous eruption, lactation and abuse of mercury. Though some of these now seem archaic (e.g. disappearance of a cutaneous eruption) others, such as joy from prosperity and wounded self-esteem, we may phrase differently now but could still be seen as possible life stressors that could trigger a manic episode.

Two French psychiatrists working in the 1850s were the first to link mania and melancholia, though they had different views on the nature of this illness. One, Falret, termed the illness *folie circulaire* which he described as a continuous cycle of mania followed by melancholia with lucid intervals in between, the prognosis of which he deemed hopeless. Baillarger described *folie à double forme* in which mania and melancholia switch into each other but there was no lucid interval between the two (Angst & Marneros, 2001). A German psychiatrist, Karl Kahlbaum, introduced the ideas of Falret and Baillarger to a German audience but in his textbook he supported Falret's conception and opposed Baillarger's (Angst & Marneros, 2001). It was another German psychiatrist, Emile Kraepelin who, building on the work of these earlier psychiatrists, attempted to develop systematic clinical descriptions of the major mental disorders and, in doing so, differentiate between mood disorders and psychotic disorders. It was he that described what we would now call schizophrenia as 'dementia praecox' because he saw it as an illness with a chronic deteriorating course. He separately described an illness that had periodic insanity and episodes of melancholia and this he termed 'manic-depressive insanity'. This illness had a relapsing and remitting course and was not prone, in most cases, to lead to dementia. The prevailing view at that time was that madness led, in most cases, to a chronic state of mental enfeeblement. It has been suggested (Hare, 1981) that

Kraepelin was able to identify a group of mental health issues that didn't lead to dementia because gradual improvements in the general physical health of the populations in many countries across Europe in the latter part of the nineteenth century meant people started to live longer and were not so physically enfeebled in older age, positively affecting the course of various mental disorders.

Kraepelin's conception of manic depression included within it all types of depressive illnesses and so included a very heterogeneous set of conditions. This muddied the waters concerning what exactly manic depression was. Psychiatrists in other parts of Europe, especially Scandinavia and France, disagreed strongly with Kraepelin's construct and so the term did not gain wide usage for many years (Angst & Marneros, 2001). It was during the 1950s that researchers began to look again at the differences between unipolar depression and a disorder that included periods of both depressive and manic phases. This was partly stimulated by the finding of the effectiveness of lithium to treat the bipolar subgroup of the manic-depressive cohort (Healy, 2010).

The term *bipolar* first appeared as a diagnostic category in the third revision of the American Psychiatric Association's Diagnostic and Statistical manual (DSM-III) which appeared in 1980. It then became incorporated in the European diagnostic manual the International Classification of Diseases in its tenth revision (ICD-10) in 1992. In recent years the advent of more drugs to treat bipolar disorder, and the licensing of some antipsychotics to treat it, has led to more research and a broadening of the concept of bipolar disorder into a continuum of manic conditions (Angst & Marneros, 2001). This means that a concept that started broad and as 'mania' becoming narrower with the concept of 'manic depression' has now broadened out again as it has become conceptualised as a spectrum disorder.

Due to its association with creativity and genius, bipolar disorder is a much more attractive label than most others in the mental health lexicon. This means, unsurprisingly, that many people with significant mental health issues would rather have a diagnosis of bipolar disorder than other mental health conditions (Chan & Sireling, 2010). Research (Ruggero et al., 2010) has shown that, due to some shared characteristics such as affective instability, clinicians

sometimes misdiagnose people with emotionally unstable personality disorder (EUPD) as having bipolar disorder. Furthermore, the
inclusion of bipolar II disorder in the bipolar spectrum, for which
the person need only have had one hypomanic episode and one
episode of depression, may also provide for many false positives.
This is because research (Angst et al., 2010) has demonstrated that
elevated mood including elation, being energetic, self-confident and
extraverted is on a continuum and may represent normal 'highs'.
Sometimes people who have a tendency to be lower in mood most
of the time can misinterpret occasions when they are actually just
happy as pathological and believe themselves to be in a state of an
unnatural 'high' mood. When such people present to services with
low mood and are asked if they have ever had an episode of elevated
mood some will remember back to times when they were happy and
report it as a 'high' episode. This is one of the reasons why bipolar
II can be over inclusive in the numbers of people that attract the
diagnosis.

Causes of bipolar disorder

Findings of studies into possible structural and functional abnormalities in the brains of people with bipolar disorder have produced differing, and sometimes contradictory, results (Strakowski & Sax, 2000;
Johnson, 2003). Studies into secondary mania (see Strakowski &
Sax, 2000 for a review), i.e. mania occurring after an injury such as
a stroke, show it occurring after two types of brain injury; damage
to regions on the right side or damage to the striatum and/or thala-
mus. However, they also caution that most cases of mania occur in
people who have not had injuries to these regions. Therefore, these
regions may be implicated in the onset of mania in some cases but
these findings are only suggestive. It is thought (Miklowitz & Johnson, 2006) that dysregulation in the systems of the neurotransmitters
dopamine and serotonin interact with deficits in other neurotransmitter systems. One should be cautious when drawing conclusions as
studies of neurotransmitter metabolites remain inconclusive, though
there is some evidence of reduced activity of the inhibitory neurotransmitter gamma-aminobutyric acid (GABA) from post-mortem

studies (Linden, 2012). Studies (Miklowitz & Johnson, 2006) have shown increased activity in the amygdalas of people with bipolar disorder, a brain region which has a key role in emotional response. Though neurodevelopmental events including obstetric and prenatal events have been demonstrated to be causal factors in schizophrenia this hasn't been shown to be the case in bipolar disorder (ibid.).

Genetic studies seem to point to a familial link in bipolar disorder. This has been demonstrated via studies into monozygotic (identical) twins as they have demonstrated a higher rate of bipolar disorder than studies into non-identical twins. Environmental factors could explain some of these results, but studies into adopted twins have shown higher rates of bipolar disorder in the offspring of parents with bipolar disorder who were adopted and did not grow up with their natural parents than in the offspring of those adopted who had well biological parents (Segman & Lerer, 2000). Exactly how people inherit bipolar disorder remains unknown, no single gene has been identified as responsible and, as is the case with schizophrenia, it is highly unlikely that one will. Various models have been postulated of how genes may influence or cause a vulnerability to have a bipolar episode, the most plausible is that many genes confer a small increase in risk (Craddock & Sklar, 2013) though how they interact with each other is still unknown. Despite the evidence of a genetic component it is unlikely that genes alone explain either the onset of bipolar disorder or its subsequent course and other factors, such as early life trauma and environmental factors, are equally important.

Bipolar disorder and creativity

There has long been a view that bipolar disorder is linked to creativity. It should be noted that this may be true of the elevated 'high' phase of the disorder, however, the depressive phases with low energy levels, poor concentration, negative thoughts etc. all hamper normal functioning, never mind excelling in one's chosen field. It has been suggested however (Hershman & Lieb, 1998), that even the low moods when not too severe can be helpful as they encourage the critical judgement necessary to fine-tune the individual's particular piece of work. As Hershman and Lieb (ibid.) point out, being perceived as a genius has a dynamic quality as many societal influences including taste, fashion, knowledge and understanding all influence what and whom are seen as deserving of the mantle of genius.

The Greek philosopher Aristotle associated great ability with melancholia and throughout history many philosophers have thought that there is a link between forms of madness and genius. For example the nineteenth century French novelist (and woman), George Sand, stated that 'between genius and madness there is often not the thickness of a hair' (quoted in Hershman & Lieb, 1998). Many people have subscribed to this view probably because it adds a frisson of romance, even danger, to the 'artist' or genius as it equates their creativity with a high level of unpredictability and intense emotion. This view was persuasively contested by Anthony Storr in his fascinating book *The Dynamics of Creation* (Storr, 1993). In his book Storr argues that not all creative people are driven by some form of psychopathology but could better be thought of as 'a dynamic of the normal'. Sometimes the discovery of a talent encourages an individual down a certain path. Furthermore, such talents often become apparent in childhood and are often encouraged by the praise of parents and others. Storr (ibid.) makes the point that, even in individuals with a considerable degree of psychopathology, such as the writer Joseph Conrad, the relationship between his psychopathology and his chosen career as a writer is by no means clear and that Freud himself stated that psychoanalysis, despite its focus on people's motives for their behaviour, was unable to explain creativity. Indeed, in his article on creativity and psychopathology Felix Post (1994) studied the mental health of 291 famous men of various disciplines and found that what helped them succeed, as well as talent, was their drive, perseverance, industry and meticulousness. Post found that, though most of his subjects had unusual personality characteristics in terms of psychopathology, only depressive disorders, alcoholism and possibly psychosexual problems were more prevalent than would be expected and, of all the artistic careers, this was only found to be so in the case of writers. In a later study (Post, 1996) into the psychopathology of 100 British and American writers he found that there was a high frequency of bipolar disorder especially among poets, almost all of whom were white Anglo-Saxon Americans.

The reality of bipolar disorder is that the illness can have negative, as well as positive, effects on people's lives. The severity of the illness is the most important factor, if an individual is either so low or so 'high' that they require hospitalisation this will severely impact on their creative talents. Hershman and Lieb (1998) state that for some people it is the grandiosity associated with manic states that sustains them in their endeavours no matter what opinions other people may have and this excessive self-belief helps creative people through periods (sometimes very long ones) where they are not recognised and often endure poverty and severe hardship. Storr (1993) argues using a psychodynamic approach that the person with bipolar disorder is driven by a need to protect themselves from the danger of a loss of self-esteem. Their creative exploits, be they great works of art or literature, are a way of protecting the individual against the depression that would follow a loss of self-esteem. Interestingly in Storr's view, another way of protecting oneself is the 'manic defence' in his model and mania is a way of reversing and denying the underlying depressive personality. It is worth noting that Storr accepts that this 'manic defence' attempt to deny depression is milder than a true hypomanic or manic episode during which the individual becomes so manic that they can no longer function.

People with bipolar disorder

George III (1738–1820) was king of Great Britain from 1760 until his death. Many people today believe that King George III suffered from intermittent porphyria which is a disease that attacks the nervous system and usually causes abdominal pain, hypertension and tachycardia, but can also cause seizures and psychiatric symptoms including hallucinations. This view was proposed by the psychiatrists and historians Ida Macalpine and Richard Hunter in the 1960s and became accepted as fact. However, recent researchers have questioned this, pointing out that even when this argument was put forward some experts in porphyria disagreed (Peters & Beveridge, 2010). A review of King George III's extensive medical records and contemporary diaries of courtiers and equerries led Peters and Beveridge (ibid.) to argue that he experienced four or five periods of mania. It appears that these episodes of illness occurred at times of significant historical events including the American War of Independence, the Irish Rebellion and the French Revolutionary and Napoleonic Wars. As people with bipolar disorder are very sensitive to stressful situations it is therefore possible that these historically challenging events provoked relapses in his manic illness. To treat his first episode of mania, in 1788 his new physician Francis Willis stopped all the lancing, cupping and blistering that had been performed on the king up until that point and instead controlled his activities and used a quasi-mesmerising technique of fixing the patient with his eye, Willis also stressed the importance of adequate nutrition (Peters & Willis, 2013).

During his first well-documented episode of illness in 1788, the king did suffer from abdominal pain similar to what can happen with porphyria, however, he then developed what appears to be a full manic episode. He exhibited pressure of speech and flight of ideas, jumping rapidly from one topic to another. He also became sexually disinhibited (Peters & Beveridge, 2010), another symptom common in periods of elevated mood. When he was at his worst the king was put in his strait waistcoat and restraining chair. This episode lasted from October 1788 to March 1789, by which time the king became much calmer and more rational. Francis Willis's son, Dr Thomas Willis, met with the king regularly over the next 12 years and the Willis family remained involved in his care throughout the rest of his life.

King George had several episodes of mania from which he recovered until his final episode in 1810 (from which he did not recover) and he remained ill for the last ten years of his life. It is thought this episode was triggered by the death of one of his daughters. This extended period of illness incapacitated the king and led to the establishment of a regency with his son, the Prince of Wales, being placed as regent to act in his place. Peters and Beveridge (ibid.) argue that the acute manic episodes King George III experienced were of a length that one would expect in bipolar disorder, they also note that physical illnesses can often co-occur with bipolar disorder and they conclude that the evidence for bipolar disorder is stronger than that for porphyria.

Sir Isaac Newton (1643–1727) was a scientist with interests in many fields including mathematics, physics and astronomy. In 1705 he was one of the first scientists to be knighted (by Queen Anne). Storr (1993) believes that Newton had a schizoid personality and points to his lack of interest in personal relationships, his emotional detachment and his solitary nature. Others such as Keynes (2008) believe that his main episode of illness was due to mercury poisoning. However, there is strong evidence of Newton being emotionally labile that contradicts the view of him being consistently emotionally detached. As a young man he listed all his childhood sins and these included threatening to burn his stepfather and mother along with the house they were in. He was also known to have fits of rage that led to him verbally abusing the family servants and his siblings. At university he worked excessively long hours and slept little, which could be indicative of a manic temperament. Hershman and Lieb (1998) point to a pattern that existed throughout his scientific career of manic inspiration and tireless work that sometimes transitioned into depressive episodes that interfered with the completion of his work. They also believe that the social isolation he exhibited was related to his depressive episodes rather than a schizoid nature. As he got older, there is evidence that Newton became more distant from people and more sensitive to those that disagreed with him. This mistrust of others tipped over into a full paranoid episode in 1693; at that time he was over active, did not sleep for days and wrote letters to his friends accusing them of plotting against him (Storr, 1993). After this episode subsided Newton became low in mood and wrote to his friends apologising for his accusatory letters. He had several other depressive episodes in his life but never another episode of outright mania and paranoia. It isn't thought that Newton received any medical help for his paranoia.

William Pitt the Elder (1708–1778) was prime minister of Britain from 1766 to 1768. He was apparently a brilliant orator and debater. His criticisms of careerist politicians and corruption made him popular with the general public. At one point he held the post of Paymaster General to the forces, a position that the holder generally used as an opportunity for corruption to make themselves wealthy but Pitt only took his official salary. Pitt came from a wealthy and influential family but one that had a strong history of mental health problems.

Both his grandfather and father had reputations for being explosive and impulsive characters and one of his sisters was committed to, and died in, a mental hospital.

Pitt experienced depressive episodes of considerable length one lasted between 1751 and 1754 (Davidson, 2011). At other times he was impulsive, exhibited rapid energy, great self-confidence and was impulsively extravagant with money, often putting himself into debt: traits very common in people who are to a certain degree hypomanic. These traits were of great service to his country from 1754 onwards during what became known as The Seven Years War, throughout which, though not officially the prime minister, he effectively assumed the leadership of government. He suffered from what he himself called 'gout in the brain' from 1765 and admitted to major mental health issues. These had not resolved when he became prime minister in 1766 and Davidson (ibid.) states that he had severe depression but with manic elements that made it difficult for him to function and his government was effectively leaderless for significant periods of time. He isolated himself from others, sitting in a darkened room refusing food and weeping, yet at the same time devising grandiose plans to enlarge his country home by 34 bedrooms even though he lacked the finances to attempt this (ibid.). He tendered his resignation from the government in 1768 due to his poor health. Pitt collapsed in the House of Lords in April 1778 while debating how to conclude the War of Independence with America and died a month later.

The composer Beethoven will be discussed elsewhere in relation to his duel diagnosis of bipolar disorder and alcoholism. Similar to Newton, he would become so driven by his moods and focussed on his work that he would forget to eat and would work late in to the night until his work was finished. It has been suggested (Hershman & Lieb, 1998; Forster, 2012) that the famous author Charles Dickens had bipolar disorder due to his driven quality and periods of great energy. One thing that Dickens and Beethoven had in common was there habit of attempting to control their excess energy by going on very long walks. Dickens would walk throughout the night in London and later published a book of his walks; similarly Beethoven would compose as he walked for hours in the country side. Also like Newton, Beethoven was prone to irritability and suspiciousness, this would have increased as he became increasingly deaf as there is a strong correlation between deafness and paranoia. Beethoven's numerous depressive episodes were well documented and he often found it difficult to attend to his self-care and often looked dishevelled; during these periods he found it difficult to work and he ruminated on whether or not to commit suicide (Dehm, 2008).

Politics can be a very stressful occupation and itself can lead to mental health difficulties as has been discussed with the British politician David Lloyd George. Like Lloyd George the nineteenth century British politician, William Ewart Gladstone (1809–1898) often experienced physical illnesses when stressed. For people with a mental illness the stress of political life can often provoke a relapse and it seems that Gladstone experienced hypomanic episodes often followed by depression on a number of occasions while a major political figure (Davidson, 2011). In total he served as prime minister for 12 years over four separate periods in office. When he left office for the last time in 1894 he was, at 84, the oldest person to serve as prime minister. Davidson (ibid.) estimated that Gladstone experienced at least 15 episodes of depression often preceded by periods of elevated mood during which he was irritable, impulsive, overspent and exhibited pressure of speech, all of which are indicative of hypomania. Impulsivity is not a good quality to possess when one is the political leader of a major power. Gladstone did at times make impulsive decisions, for example, he dissolved parliament suddenly in 1874. This left little time to campaign between the dissolution of parliament and the general election and, despite the timing of the election being of his choosing, his ill-prepared Liberal party lost to the Conservatives.

Gladstone did seek the help of doctors and took rest cures, however, at other times he was able to pull himself out of his episodes of depression by focusing on his work and, like many others in the age before any modern treatments (be they pharmacological or talking therapies), he dealt with his mental health issues by sheer force of his personality. One thing he did for many years to control his considerable energy was excessive tree felling on his country estate, something he continued to do until he was 82 and which Davidson (ibid.) suggests came close to ridding it of all trees! Like Darwin and Dickens he also went on very long walks, one of which was 33 miles in length. One of the other activities he engaged in, that could be seen as impulsive and could possibly have put himself in danger of blackmail, was his rescue work with prostitutes. This he did from around 1849 onwards. He would, after a long session in the House of Commons, go out late into the night meeting prostitutes. By 1854 he estimated he had spoken to between 80 and 90 prostitutes (Matthew, 1997) in an attempt to encourage them to give up prostitution and take up other forms of work. Though this work was well meaning on one level, on another there was obviously a sexual element to it, as he noted that from 1849 onwards he began flogging himself to counter the stimulation he had felt from meeting these women (this self-flagellation was known as the 'English Vice' in the nineteenth century) (ibid.). He was eventually the victim of a blackmail attempt due to his nocturnal activities in 1853 but he went to the police over it and, despite warnings from friends, continued his work with prostitutes sometimes staying long into the night at their homes despite being aware of how this must look to others. This activity, though understandable on one level as a moral act, also seems due to its extent and longevity to have been something of a compulsion he found difficult to break. This is clear from the fact that he felt guilty for doing it and often flogged himself after his meetings (ibid.). It seems that Gladstone used his heavy workload, tree felling and long walks to control his hypomanic episodes and his flogging to control his heightened sexual urges, he managed a very successful political career and he died at home at the age of 88.

Like politicians, people in the Arts are also well represented in the history of bipolar disorder. The actress Vivien Leigh (1913–1967) saw her career and marriage to Laurence Olivier blighted by her illness. She would have days of being irritable, unpredictable and overactive that would then be followed by longer episodes of low mood (Strachan, 2018). As with many people, her episodes of illness were precipitated by the stress in her life. As an actress she appeared in many high profile films such as *Gone with the Wind* and *A Streetcar Named Desire* which were stressful to make, requiring long hours of work and separation from her friends and family. She also appeared on the stage often and was sensitive to poor reviews which did occur on occasion. Furthermore, she suffered a miscarriage in 1945 which precipitated a major breakdown, though it is thought that this wasn't her first episode of illness. She had a number of episodes of illness and was treated with ECT on several occasions, a treatment that as discussed earlier is still used today at times for people who are severely depressed. Unfortunately, her illness impacted on her acting career and she made far fewer films than she should have. Tragically she died of tuberculosis at the young age of 53.

These days, people who experience bipolar disorder have a wider range of treatment options than Vivien Leigh's doctors had available to them. Among them is Kay Redfield Jamison, the American psychologist, academic and Professor of Psychiatry who has written extensively on bipolar disorder. Her book, *An Unquiet Mind*, is her memoire of living with bipolar disorder and in it she discusses what treatments she has found helpful. At the age of 30 she attempted suicide by taking a massive overdose of lithium. She discusses how, if she had the choice, would she chose to have the illness and says that 'yes' she would as it has meant she has had more experiences, felt emotions more intensely and that this intensity of thoughts and emotions has forced on her new perspectives on life and has tested the very limits of her mind (Redfield Jamison, 1996). She acknowledges the support of her family, friends, colleagues and doctors in helping her when she was ill but also notes the positive effect that the drug lithium has had on her illness and often advocates on the treatability of the illness. Redfield Jamison has also written a biography of the Pulitzer Prize winning poet Robert Lowell who was open about his bipolar disorder and in it she reviews his medical records. This includes fascinating details about his episodes of illness and, like Redfield Jamison, Lowell also took lithium to try to control his mood swings.

Other contemporary figures such as Stephen Fry and Carrie Fisher have also made great efforts to challenge the stigma that accompanies mental health difficulties by speaking out about their own experiences. Stephen Fry made the two-part television documentary *The Secret Life of the Manic Depressive* in 2006. This was a frank and fascinating discussion of his experiences with bipolar disorder. He discusses how he became suicidal in 1995 after a bad review of his performance in the play *Cell Mates*. He describes going into his garage, sealing the door with a duvet and sitting in his car for at least two hours with his hands on the ignition key in what was a serious consideration of committing suicide. Instead, he decided he could no longer live in England and so fled to Europe before returning to England where he was subsequently diagnosed with bipolar disorder. He has since written about it extensively and is candid about how disruptive he was when he was younger and before he was diagnosed. Fry was expelled from his school for his disruptive behaviour and, with hindsight, thinks that his illness began when he was 14. At 17 he impulsively stole a credit card and spent three months on remand. At the time he made the programmes he stated that he still experienced three to four depressive episodes per year.

Stephen Fry was interviewed by the Bafta winning actor Adam Deacon for a BBC news report in 2016, Deacon himself was diagnosed with bipolar disorder after a breakdown. They both agreed that the prevalence of social media can be dangerous for people with bipolar disorder as the impulsivity that sometimes accompanies bipolar disorder, especially in the manic phase, means that people may take to social media and post things that they later regret. Deacon himself was found guilty of harassment after making a threat to a colleague over twitter while unwell; eventually he was detained in hospital under the Mental Health Act. He was admitted as manic and paranoid but a combination of being removed from his stressful life, talking to staff and other service users and medication helped him recover in three weeks.

In the first part of his documentary on manic depression Stephen Fry described Carrie Fisher (1956–2016) the American actor as the poster child for manic depression. Like Fry, she was open and honest about her illness and struggles with addiction helping to challenge the stigma associated with both. He interviewed her and she described 'highs' of her manic phases as better than any drug you could ever do. Elsewhere she has described having bipolar disorder since the age of 24 but refusing to accept the diagnosis or any help until she was 28. She was open about her alcohol and drug misuse and stated that she used painkillers to try to calm her elevated moods. Fisher also talked about going to AA meetings for her alcohol problem, using group therapy and having ECT to treat her bipolar disorder. On the issue of creativity, Fisher stated that when her mood was elevated she felt that she was more talented even though this wasn't necessarily true. She talked frankly about not sleeping for six days and becoming delusional. In the second part, Fry spoke to the award winning actor Richard Dreyfus who spoke about his bipolar illness and how mood stabilisers such as lithium have helped him.

Treatment of bipolar disorder

The most effective pharmacological treatment for bipolar disorder is the alkali metal *lithium*, a compound version of which is often known as lithium salts. This has been used as a treatment for various conditions, including gout, since the nineteenth century. Its use as a medication for mental health also has a long history, mineral springs containing lithium had a reputation as 'crazy waters' (Shorter, 2009). The British physician Alfred Baring Garrod was the first to confirm that gout was caused by an excess of uric acid in 1847 and he used lithium to treat it. He also thought that an excess of uric acid caused depression (what was sometimes called 'brain gout') and he recommended the use of lithium for depression. It was first prescribed for mania in 1871 in New York and for depression in Denmark near the end of the nineteenth century (ibid.). However, these early pioneering uses were largely forgotten until John Cade used it in 1949 in Melbourne Australia. Cade thought that toxic factors associated with uric acid caused psychosis and, in an attempt to prove this, injected guinea pigs with his patients' urine – unfortunately most died immediately, however when he injected them with lithium they became calm. Based on this observation he treated a number of his manic patients with lithium; though his hypothesis was incorrect, lithium did work very well for a number of his patients. Unfortunately, due to the then unknown toxic effects lithium can have, one of his patients died and Cade then stopped using it (Bourgeois & Masson, 2017). Unfortunately for Cade, as he published his findings on lithium's positive effects in an Australian journal it did not have the impact it should have had and he did not get much recognition for several years. His study was picked up by Danish psychiatrists in the early 1950s and Mogens Schou conducted a randomised controlled trial that proved its effectiveness for mania. However, due to risks associated with its toxicity, it wasn't until 1958 (Shorter, 2009) when reliable methods of measuring the blood concentration of lithium were developed that it became widespread.

Despite its proven effectiveness the mechanisms by which it acts as a mood stabiliser are poorly understood. It is known that it works on multiple levels, from the macroscopic anatomy to microscopic intracellular signalling (Malhi et al., 2013). There are changes in brain structure associated with lithium use. Increased volume of the anterior cingulate cortex, the ventral prefrontal cortex, the hippocampus and the amygdala – structures involved in emotional regulation – have been reported (ibid.). At the neurotransmitter level, lithium modulates dopamine, glutamate and GABA neurotransmission (ibid.). Adverse effects on kidney and thyroid function are common. Management must include monitoring of the serum level, kidney function and thyroid function. From the 1990s onwards other drugs have been marketed as 'mood stabilisers' and these have usually been anticonvulsants or compounds closely related to anticonvulsants which may also hint at their putative mode of action.

Using a historical epidemiological approach, Harris et al. (2005) demonstrated that, compared to a hundred year period before its introduction, the advent of lithium and other mood stabilisers had led to better management of acute episodes of illness with shorter stays in hospital. Interestingly, they also found that the use of mood stabilisers did not reduce the time to the next relapse or the number of relapses that occurred concluding that their research indicates that there is no room for complacency in clinical practice. Antidepressants are usually used when people are clinically depressed, however, when people have bipolar disorder care must be taken when prescribing antidepressants as they can sometimes elevate the mood too far and precipitate a hypomanic episode. This can make treating the low moods that are a major part of bipolar disorder difficult in some people.

It has been argued (Lam et al., 1999) that, due to the initial reported success of lithium, other therapies including talking therapies were neglected. This, the authors argue, is surprising given the fact that stress can often trigger relapses in bipolar disorder and so teaching people how to deal with life stressors is important. People should be offered the same therapies that are used for major depressive episodes including interpersonal therapy (IPT), cognitive behavioural therapy (CBT) and other therapies with proven efficacy in depression. CBT seems to have more effect on the depressive part of bipolar disorder than on mania (Lam et al., 2005). For bipolar disorder psychosocial interventions should be used in conjunction with medication and structured individual, group or family therapies that have proven efficacy in bipolar disorder should be used. Family therapy interventions have been found to be effective with people with schizophrenia and similar approaches have been used for people with bipolar disorder. Studies (Miklowitz & Johnson, 2006) have shown that a family intervention that included psychoeducation, communication enhancement training and problem-solving skills reduced rates of relapse and rehospitalisation. Psychoeducation should aim to help people identify the warning signs of an impending relapse, for example, for many people one of the first symptoms of relapse is a broken sleep pattern, at this point people may want to make sure that they get adequate sleep if they can or may want to address whatever stressors are impacting on their ability to sleep. People should be made aware of their own individual risk factors for relapse – for some that may be overwork, life stressors, illicit drug or alcohol misuse, or non-compliance with medication.

In conclusion, we can see that bipolar disorder can devastate people's lives and is associated with high rates of suicide. However, it is also true that many people are able to live fulfilling lives often with a combination of medication, supportive social networks, therapeutic interventions and the help of mental health services. Creativity may be associated with bipolar disorder but bipolar disorder is as likely to happen to a bus driver as a Beethoven and, whether Beethoven's work was positively or negatively affected if at all by his bipolar disorder, is open to debate. The important thing is that help is out there for people in many parts of the world and with that help many people can recover and live meaningful lives.

7

Dual Diagnosis

According to the UK mental health charity Mind, the term *dual diagnosis* was first used in the United States in the 1980s to describe people with a psychotic illness who also used illicit drugs and/or alcohol (Phillips & Labrow, 2004). Since that time the term has become increasingly prevalent in clinical practice. The meaning of dual diagnosis has also been broadened to include individuals who have both a mental disorder, such as schizophrenia or clinical depression, and concurrent alcohol and/or recreational or prescription drug dependency. There are also examples of people with more than one mental health difficulty though these are rarely considered to be dual diagnoses in clinical practice; for example anxiety and depression often co-occur but this would not be thought of as a dual diagnosis and the usual practice would be to treat both concurrently.

Often people take alcohol, prescription or recreational drugs to deal with the symptoms of their illness and this is termed 'self-medicating' by some clinicians. It isn't surprising that when people are feeling anxious or stressed they take substances that help to calm them down. The problem is that, although in the short term these substances can seem helpful, over time they can have a number of negative effects including, dependence, withdrawal symptoms, problems in relationships, difficulty functioning in day-to-day tasks and they can sometimes cause other mental health problems. An example of this is the case of Miles Davis the jazz musician, he used cocaine and barbiturates to deal with the pain caused by his sickle cell anaemia, unfortunately this resulted in psychotic episodes in which he became paranoid and experienced auditory hallucinations

(Wills, 2003) which severely affected his ability to perform and he hardly played his trumpet for five years.

The World Health Organization points out that mental health issues and substance abuse issues are common in all regions of the world, however, approximately 75 per cent of people in low-income countries have no access to treatments for them. They hope to address this via the Mental Health Gap Action Programme (mhGAP) which hopes to scale up services in lower-income countries (WHO, 2017c). An example of this is the WHO designed QualityRights initiative that is reforming mental health services and promoting human rights in various parts of the world. One such initiative has taken place in the state of Gujarat in India where this approach has helped to change the model from a purely symptom-focussed biomedical model to a more social one based on human rights and recovery. As part of this approach, people with lived experience of mental health problems have taken on peer support roles. These voluntary positions are helpful not only to the service users but also to the volunteers as they give them a sense of purpose and help raise their self-esteem.

Ludwig van Beethoven (1770–1827) is one of the world's most famous composers. It is also well-documented that he experienced a number of depressive episodes and a smaller number of episodes of elation which, combined, could indicate he possibly suffered from bipolar disorder. He had low tolerance levels and would often become angry with people sometimes coming to blows. It has been argued that his moodiness is reflected in his music, even that the sudden changes in tempo in some pieces is reflective of his bipolar moods (Mai, 2008). As an indication of his impulsiveness, Beethoven lived at 24 different addresses between 1792 and 1824, often moving lodgings due to falling out with his neighbours or landlords. It is well known that Beethoven went deaf in his late 20s, it is also well-documented that alongside his mood disorder he drank alcohol very heavily. Beethoven suffered from a number of physical ailments, unfortunately his tempestuous nature meant he often fell out with his physicians and he had at least 11 different ones; a number of whom advised him to moderate his alcohol consumption. He died aged 56 and his autopsy found severe liver damage which was probably related to his alcohol abuse. His last words reported were 'pity,

pity, too late' after hearing he was being sent a case of wine which he knew he was too ill to ever taste.

The writer Edgar Allan Poe (1809–1849), famous for macabre stories such as *The Raven* and *The Pit and the Pendulum*, also experienced a number of mental health issues including depression and mood swings. Poe had certainly experienced adversity in his life: his father left the family when he was one and his mother died of tuberculosis when he was only two. He was taken in by a family but became estranged from them when he went to university and ran up huge gambling debts. At the age of 26 he married his first cousin when she was only 13, the nature of their relationship remains subject to speculation. Unfortunately, like his mother, she died of tuberculosis at the young age of 24. Poe, alongside his mental health issues, also drank heavily and after his wife died he was jailed for public intoxication. He also experienced visual hallucinations of his dead wife in which she was being dismembered (Giammarco, 2013). Sadly, Poe died young at the age of 40 and in mysterious circumstances. He was found in, or near, a tavern in a confused state uttering the phrase 'Reynolds, Oh Reynolds!' repeatedly and suffering from visual hallucinations, he then slipped into a coma and died days later. The cause of death given was 'congestion of the brain' due to hepatic encephalopathy caused by alcoholism. Various other theories have arisen as to the cause of his death, the most interesting of which is that he was a victim of 'cooping'. This was a practice in America in which gangs would grab vulnerable adults when an election was immanent, keep them in a room (the coop) sometimes for days, mistreat them, ply them with alcohol and make them go around the city voting multiple times for a candidate. This theory arose with Poe because he had been missing for several days, turned up on the day of an election, was obviously distressed and the clothes he was wearing didn't fit him. This fitted the cooping theory because the gangs would often change the clothes of their victims to disguise them so that they could vote multiple times.

At a similar time in England lived the poet and artist Dante Gabriel Rossetti (1828–1882). Rossetti was one of the founders of the Pre-Raphaelite Brotherhood. There were mental health problems in his family, his father suffered from depressive episodes as did his younger sister the poet Christina Rossetti famous for poems such as

Goblin Market and the Christmas poem (later turned into a hymn), *In the Bleak Midwinter*. Rossetti was well known for relationships with his models, his first wife Elizabeth Siddall had been one of his models, she was always quite a frail person and prone to both physical illness and depressive episodes. In 1862 at the age of 32 she died from an overdose of laudanum (a powerful and addictive opioid painkiller). This affected Rossetti badly, possibly partly through guilt that he had had numerous affairs with his models while she was alive. After a complicated affair with the wife of his friend William Morris and bad reactions to his first published collection of poetry, Rossetti had become dependent on alcohol and chloral hydrate (a sedative). The abuse of drugs and alcohol plus his depressive illness provoked a psychotic illness and he became paranoid and experienced hallucinations. His brother William sought medical help and, though he did take an overdose in an attempt to commit suicide, with the care of friends he did partially recover. Unfortunately, his physical health deteriorated further and he became reclusive dying of kidney disease at the age of 53.

The American playwright Tennessee Williams (1911–1983) who wrote some of the major post-war American plays including *A Streetcar Named Desire* and *Cat on a Hot Tin Roof*, was prone to depressive episodes. As mentioned earlier in Chapter 5, his sister Rose had developed schizophrenia and underwent a disastrous lobotomy leaving her institutionalised for the rest of her life. This affected Williams and he was terrified of also becoming 'mad', this fear probably contributed to his bouts of depression. As he got older his alcohol and drug use spiralled. This wasn't helped by his own doctor treating his depression with ever-larger doses of amphetamines. The drugs and alcohol severely reduced his talent and his later plays were not as well received. Tragically, Williams choked to death on a plastic bottle cap at the age of 71. Williams was in good company as a writer with a dual diagnosis – Ernest Hemmingway was also an alcoholic and experienced depressive episodes and Hunter S. Thompson used copious amounts of drugs and alcohol and, like Hemmingway, died by shooting himself.

The Pulitzer Prize winning poet Anne Sexton (1928–1974) had a very different trajectory towards dual diagnosis. After a difficult upbringing she married young and seems to have developed mental health problems as a young adult. She had lots of therapy and it was her psychiatrist that encouraged her to write poetry to help with her mood. Her first book was called *To Bedlam and Part Way Back* and told of her struggles with her mental health and her time in mental health hospitals. One of the poems, *Wanting to Die*, addresses her experiences of being suicidal and is considered by many one her best poems. Despite her growing fame she found it difficult to cope with the demands of life and her depressive episodes. By the late 1960s she was using alcohol excessively and, as with other creative individuals, the alcohol affected the quality of her work. Though she had a significant amount of therapy throughout her adult life she seemed to spiral out of control, the alcohol obviously didn't help. Sadly she ended her life by carbon monoxide poisoning at the age of 45. After her death there were claims she had had an affair with one of her psychiatrists which, given her vulnerable state, would only had adversely affected her further. Another therapist gave the tape recordings of her therapy sessions to an author for their biography of Sexton which was very controversial as this was a breach of trust and many have argued these tapes should have remained confidential.

As with dementia, the adverse effects of alcohol and drugs should be a concern to us when the individuals using them are occupying positions of power since they can adversely affect the individual's judgement and decision making. A number of British prime ministers have had a combination of a mental health problem and a dependency on drugs and or alcohol – Pitt the Younger (1759–1806), despite being recognised as a very successful prime minister, had a serious alcohol problem as well as an anxiety disorder; the Earl of Rosebery (1847–1929), prone both to anxiety and depression, was known to take both morphine and an alcohol derivative, sulphonal (Davidson, 2011), it is thought he even tried to enliven his speeches in parliament by taking cocaine before he spoke, the cocktail of the three drugs apparently made his speeches quite shambolic at times.

Much has been written about Churchill's mood, his dementia and his considerable consumption of alcohol – he had his first whisky of the day after breakfast, his glass was rarely empty after that, and he had champagne with lunch and dinner (ibid.). He had to be led away from the House of Commons on occasions when too drunk to complete a speech and, in 1944 during the Second World War, turned up drunk to a Defence Committee meeting and wanted to commence poison gas attacks on German cities, which was only prevented by an intervention by the Chiefs of Staff. Clearly his alcohol consumption at times affected his judgement and impaired his ability to lead the nation at a time of war. An equally worrying case is that of Anthony Eden (1897–1977) who was prime minister between 1955 and 1957, a period that included the second Arab–Israeli War also often described as the Suez Crisis. This occurred when the president of Egypt, Nasser, nationalised the Suez Canal. Britain, a country that held a controlling interest in the canal, took the decision to join forces with Israel and France, invade Egypt and attempt to depose Nasser. At the time Prime Minister Eden, prone to anxiety and poor sleep, was taking barbiturates to help him sleep and Benzedrine (an amphetamine) to help pick him up in the morning (ibid.). Coupled with his heavy alcohol use, this combination made Eden reckless, impulsive and impaired his judgement on how to handle the crisis – according to a number of contemporary sources he became obsessed with destroying Nasser. Under American pressure, Eden was forced to call a ceasefire having only captured 23 miles of the canal. Humiliated, and with his physical health failing, Eden resigned as prime minister the following January.

Treatments for dual diagnosis

Alastair Campbell, the former Downing Street press secretary, has spoken openly about how he had a significant alcohol problem as well as a depressive illness. He has written a novel entitled *All in the Mind* that covers mental illness and alcoholism and has admitted that it is partly autobiographical. Campbell has successfully sought help for both his mood and his alcohol problem. He is a passionate campaigner for mental health causes and has described how coming to the sudden realisation that he had a drink problem was the most important thing that helped him become abstinent. He also visits his doctor for support when he notices his mood lowering. This seems to be very important for people with more than one condition seeking support for both because if they only seek support for one, such as depression, then this is likely to only be partially successful at best as the other condition, such as alcohol (a known depressant), will undermine the effectiveness of any treatment. Another person that found this to be the case was the American comedian and actor Robin Williams (1951–2014). Williams was famous for both his stand-up comedy and his many film roles. Williams had ongoing struggles with depression and with addictions to cocaine in the 1970s and 1980s and later to alcohol. He admitted himself to treatment centres several times to treat his addictions and was successful in spending many years sober between relapses. He was another person who found exercise, especially cycling, helpful in managing his low mood. Tragically, though he had been doing well and working on several films prior to his death he became very low in mood, anxious and paranoid secondary to developing Lewy body dementia and took his own life in august 2014.

Like mental health problems in general, addictions to alcohol and or illicit drugs also attract stigma. A non-judgemental approach to working with people with coexisting conditions is vital to help build trust. The use of illicit drugs can make diagnosis difficult, for example, some drugs such as amphetamines and cannabis can provoke psychotic symptoms such as paranoia and it is sometimes difficult to ascertain whether the symptoms are part of an illness onset or provoked by substances. This is particularly the case in younger people as many mental health problems, such as schizophrenia, begin in young adulthood which is also a time when many people experiment with alcohol and drugs. As alcohol is a known depressant this can also make it difficult to measure accurately how depressed a person is if they are consuming large quantities of alcohol. Furthermore, the symptoms of alcohol withdrawal are very similar to anxiety symptoms; which makes differentiating between the two conditions very difficult. Taking an inadequate history from a person where drug use is over looked could lead to a miss diagnosis of schizophrenia in an individual that only experiences psychotic symptoms while under the influence of illicit drugs. Often in developed countries with good health care systems people may be jointly worked by mental health services and substance misuse services, unfortunately such services are not always available worldwide. They are important because their roles, though complimentary, are different – the worker from the substance misuse service may be a former user of substances themselves and will aim to achieve harm reduction, reduce stigma and social exclusion, this differs from mental health services where there is a greater emphasis on the mental health issues and, in some services, achieving abstinence from the addictive substance.

Treatments for the mental health issue are the same as those described in Chapters 1, 2, 5 and 6 in this book. For the treatment of the substance misuse various talking therapies are used when available, with motivational interviewing being a well-established approach. For substance addictions the treatment differs with the substance, for example, with amphetamines the aim may be to encourage abstinence or as little use as possible whereas, for opioid dependence, many services prescribe drugs such as methadone or buprenorphine to be used as a maintenance dose and alternative to opioids.

People with both a mental health issue and a substance misuse issue have difficulties in functioning in many areas of life, this means they often present in a chaotic way and may have issues with criminal justice, benefits, housing and personal relationships. Therefore the role of the worker is to try to help support them to function effectively in these areas too. As with other areas of mental health the philosophy of the recovery model, where one aims to engender a sense of hope and optimism in the person with a dual diagnosis, is vital. Helping people take control of their addictions empowers people and helps both with their mental health issue and with other areas of their lives; this builds their resilience and helps them to make changes in their lives for the better.

Conclusion

The purpose of this book has been to describe some of the main mental health conditions that people face today. Mental health and mental ill health are part of the human condition and, as has been described, they have been with us throughout history. They are also global phenomena affecting people all around the world. That the WHO (WHO, 2018a) estimated such large percentages of people in low- and middle-income countries with mental disorders receive no treatment for their disorder and that, in high-income countries, up to half of people receive no care highlights how much still needs to be done before mental health comes anywhere near to achieving parity of esteem with physical care. Obviously, in some countries poverty and a lack of resources play a major role in preventing help being available. Views on mental health also vary across cultures and this also affects both the perception of the person with the condition and the types of care and treatment offered to them.

This book has used case studies and vignettes of many people who have experienced difficulties with their mental health, as this has enabled me to describe how real people, at various points in history, have dealt with these difficulties. It has also allowed a discussion of how perceptions of mental health conditions have evolved through time and how treatment approaches have changed. That there are still survivor movements of people who believe that mental health services have not helped them demonstrates that we should not be complacent. As history has shown on many occasions, people have believed that the care and treatment they have offered to others is the best available only for it to be superseded and rendered obsolete by subsequent generations. We must always strive to do better.

References

Abraham, S. (2016) *Eating Disorders,* 7th edition. Oxford: Oxford University Press.

Achtler, N. (2008) Hitler's Hysteria: War Neurosis and Mass Psychology in Ernst Weiß's Der Augenzeuge. *The German Quarterly,* **80**: 325–349.

Agras, W. S., Walsh, B. T., Fairburn, C. G., Wilson, G. T. & Kraemer, H. C. (2000) A Multicenter Comparison of Cognitive-Behavioral Therapy and Interpersonal Psychotherapy for Bulimia Nervosa. *Archives of General Psychiatry,* **57**: 459–466.

Altamura, A. C., Camuri, G. & Dell'Osso, B. (2013) Duration of Untreated Illness and Duration of Illness in Anxiety Disorders: Assessment and Influence on Outcome. In: D.S. Baldwin & B. E. Leonard (eds) *Anxiety Disorders, Modern Trends in Pharmacopsychiatry,* vol **29**, 111–118. Basel: Karger.

American Psychiatric Association (1980) *Diagnostic and Statistical Manual of Mental Disorders,* 3rd edition. Washington, DC: American Psychiatric Association.

Angst, J. & Marneros, A. (2001) Bipolarity from Ancient to Modern Times: Conception, Birth and Re-birth. *Journal of Affective Disorders,* **67**: 3–19.

Angst, J. & Sellaro, R. (2000) Historical perspectives and natural history of bipolar disorder. *Biological Psychiatry,* **48**: 445–457.

Angst, J., Meyer, T. D., Adolfsson, R., Skeppar, P., Carta, M., Benazzi, F., Lu, R., Wu, Y., Yang, H., Yuan, C., Morselli, P., Brieger, P., Katzmann, J., Leao, I. A., Porto, J. A., Moreno, D. H., Moreno, R. A., Soares, O. T., Vieta, E. & Gamma, A. (2010) Hypomania: A Transcultural Perspective. *World Psychiatry,* **9**: 41–49.

Appignanesi, L. (2009) *Mad, Bad and Sad: A History of Women and the Mind Doctors from 1800 to the Present.* London: Virago.

Arnold, C. (2009) *Bedlam: London and its Mad.* London: Simon & Schuster.

Asmal, L. & Stein, D. J. (2009) Anxiety and Culture. In: M.M. Anthony & M.B. Stein (eds) *Oxford Handbook of Anxiety and Related Disorders,* 657–666. New York: Oxford University Press.

Ban, T.A. (2007) Fifty Years of Chlorpromazine: A Historical Perspective. *Neuropsychiatric Disease and Treatment,* **3(4)**: 495–500.

Barlow, D.H. (2004) *Anxiety and Its Disorders*. New York: The Guilford Press.

Barnes, T.R.E. (1992) Clinical Assessment of the Extrapyramidal Side Effects of Antipsychotic Drugs. *Journal of Psychopharmacology*, **6**: 214–221.

Barton, C. H. (1907) *The Story of My Childhood*. New York: Baker & Taylor.

Bauer, M. & Pfennig, A. (2005) Epidemiology of Bipolar Disorders. *Epilepsia*, **46(4)**: 8–13.

Bebbington, P., Wilkins, S., Jones, P., Foerster, A., Murray, R., Toone, B. & Lewis, S. (1993) Life Events and Psychosis: Initial Results from the Camberwell Collaborative Psychosis Study. *British Journal of Psychiatry*, **162**: 72–79.

Bebbington, P. E. & Kuipers, E. (2003) Schizophrenia and psychosocial stresses. In: S. R. Hirsch & D. Weinberger (eds) *Schizophrenia*, 2nd edition, 613–636. Oxford, UK: Blackwell Science.

Beers, C.W. (2008) *A Mind That Found Itself*. West Valley City, USA: Waking Lion Press.

Bell, R. M. (1987) *Holy Anorexia*. Chicago, IL: University of Chicago Press.

Bentall, R. P. (1999) Why There Will Never Be a Convincing Theory of Schizophrenia. In: S. Rose (ed.) *From Brains to Consciousness? Essays on the New Sciences of the Mind*, 109–136. London: Penguin.

Bentall, R. P. (2004) *Madness Explained: Psychosis and Human Nature*. London: Penguin.

Bentall, R. P. & Morrison, A. P. (2002) More Harm Than Good: The Case Against Using Antipsychotic Drugs to Prevent Severe Mental Illness. *Journal of Mental Health*, **11**: 351–356.

Berrios, G. (2008) *The History of Mental Symptoms: Descriptive Psychopathology Since the Nineteenth Century*. Cambridge, UK: Cambridge University Press. http://beyondanxietyanddepression.com/.

Bisson, J. I., Ehlers, A., Matthews, R., Pilling, S., Richards, D. & Turner, S. (2007) Psychological Treatments for Chronic Post-Traumatic Stress Disorder. *British Journal of Psychiatry*, **190**: 97–104.

Bleuler, E. (1911) *Dementia Praecox or the Group of Schizophrenias*. New York: International Universities Press.

Boller, F. & Forbes, M. A. (1998) History of Dementia and in History: An Overview. *Journal of the Neurological Sciences*, **158**: 125–133.

Bourgeois, M. L. & Masson, M. (2017) The History of Lithium in Medicine and Psychiatry. In: G. S. Malhi, M. Masson & F. Bellivier (eds) *The Science and Practice of Lithium Therapy*, 181–188. Switzerland: Springer International Publishing.

Breier, A., Schreiber, J. L., Dyer, J. & Pickar, D. (1992) Course of Illness and Predictors of Outcome in Chronic Schizophrenia: Implications for Pathophysiology. *British Journal of Psychiatry*, **161**(suppl 18): 38–43.

Brown, G. W., Monck, E. M., Carstairs, G. M. & Wing, J. K. (1962) Influence of Family Life on the Course of Schizophrenic Illness. *British Journal of Preventative and Social Medicine,* **16**: 55–68.

Bruch, H. (1973) *Eating Disorders: Obesity, Anorexia Nervosa, and the Person Within.* New York: Basic books.

Bucknill, J. C. & Tuke, D. H. (1858) *A Manual of Psychological Medicine: Containing the History, Nosology, Description, Statistics, Diagnosis, Pathology, and Treatment of Insanity.* London: John Churchill.

Bunyan, J. (2005) *Grace Abounding to the Chief of Sinners.* London: Penguin Classics.

Burton, R. (1621) *The Anatomy of Melancholy.* Oxford. http://spenserians. cath.vt.edu/TextRecord.php?action=GET&textsid=33247.

Bynum, C. W. (1988) *Holy Feast and Holy Fast: The Religious Significance of Food to Medieval Women.* California, CA: University of California Press.

Casper, R. A. (1983). On the Emergence of Bulimia Nervosa as a Syndrome: A Historical View. *International Journal of Eating Disorders,* **2**: 3–16.

Chan, D. & Sireling, L. (2010) 'I want to Be Bipolar'... a New Phenomenon. *The Psychiatrist,* **34(3)**: 103–105.

Chen, H.-F. (2003) Articulating 'Chinese Madness': A Review of the Modern Historiography of Madness in Pre-modern China. The 1st Annual Meeting, ASHM, IHP, *Academia Sinica,* 4–8 November 2003.

Chiang, H. (ed.) (2014) *Psychiatry and Chinese history.* London: Pickering & Chatto.

Clark, D. M. (1999) Panic Disorder and Social Phobia. In: D. M. Clark & C. G. Fairbairn (eds) *Science and Practice of Cognitive Behaviour Therapy,* 119–153. Oxford: Oxford University Press.

Coleridge, S. T. (1802), Dejection: An Ode, *Poetry Foundation.* https://www. poetryfoundation.org/poems/43973/dejection-an-ode.

Craddock, N. & Sklar, P. (2013) Genetics of Bipolar Disorder. *The Lancet,* 138: 1654–1662.

Craske, M. G. & Stein, M. B. (2016) Anxiety. *The Lancet, 388*: 3048–59.

Cromby, J., Harper, D. & Reavey, P. (2013) *Psychology, Mental Health and Distress.* Basingstoke: Palgrave Macmillan.

Culbert, K., Racine, S. E. & Klump, K. L. (2015) Research Review: What We Have Learned About the Causes of Eating Disorders – A Synthesis of Sociocultural, Psychological, and Biological Research. *Journal of Child Psychology and Psychiatry,* **56(11)**: 1141–1164.

Davidson, J.R.T. (2011) *Downing Street Blues: A History of Depression and Other Mental Afflictions in British Prime Ministers.* North Carolina: McFarland.

Davidson, J.T.R., Connor, K. M. & Swartz, M. (2006) Mental Illness in U.S. Presidents Between 1776 and 1974: A Review of Biographical Sources. *The Journal of Nervous and Mental Diseases,* **194**: 47–51.

Dehm M, P. (2008) Beethoven: The Man and the Madness Behind the Music. Retrieved from https://pdfs.semanticscholar.org/76d2/3b614a922 69e719291bf8aa9042512555bda.pdf?_ga=2.35341543.772383810.1554 974957–1444760821.1554974957.

Dols, M. W. (1987) Insanity and It's Treatment in Islamic Society. *Medical History,* **31**: 1–14.

Earlstein, F. (2016) *Dementia Fand Information.* New York: NRB Publishing.

Egan, M. F. & Weinberger, D. R. (1997) Neurobiology of Schizophrenia. *Current Opinion in Neurobiology,* **7**: 701–707.

Fairburn, C. G. & Harrison, P. J. (2003) Eating Disorders. *The Lancet,* **361**: 407–416.

Fallon, P. (2008) Life Events and Their Role in Onset and Relapse in Psychosis, Research Utilising Semi-Structured Interview Methods a Literature Review. *Journal of Psychiatric and Mental Health Nursing,* **15**: 386–392.

Forster, A. (2012) Why Charles Dickens Would Be Diagnosed as Bipolar. Retrieved from www.standard.co.uk/news/london/why-charles-dickens-would-be-diagnosed-as-bipolar-8152375.html.

Fowles, D. C. (1992) Schizophrenia: Diathesis-Stress Revisited. *Annual Review of Psychology,* **43**: 303–336.

Fraguas, D. & Breathnach, C. S. (2009) Problems with Retrospective Studies of the Presence of Schizophrenia. *History of Psychiatry,* **20(1)**: 61–71.

Frith, D. (2001) *Silence of the Heart Cricket Suicides.* Edinburgh: Mainstream Publishing.

Gavett, B. E., Stern, R. A. & McKee, A. C. (2011) Chronic Traumatic Encephalopathy: A Potential Late Effect of Sport-Related Concussive and Subconcussive Head Trauma. *Clinics in Sports Medicine,* **30(1)**: 179–188.

Geddes, J. R. & Lawrie, S. M. (1995). Obstretric Complications and Schizophrenia: A Meta-Analysis. *British Journal of Psychiatry,* **167**: 786–793.

Giammarco, E. (2013) Edgar Allan Poe: A Psychological Profile. *Personality and Individual Differences,* **54**: 3–6.

Gilbert, R.E. (2003) *The Tormented President: Calvin Coolidge, Death, and Clinical Depression* (Contributions in American history) Westport, CT: Praeger.

Giordano, S. (2005) *Understanding Eating Disorders: Conceptual and Ethical Issues in the Treatment of Anorexia and Bulimia Nervosa.* Oxford: Oxford University Press.

Goedert, M. (2009) Oskar Fischer and the Study of Dementia. *Brain,* **132(4)**: 1102–1111.

Gold, J. H. (1998) Gender Differences in Psychiatric Illness and Treatments a Critical Review. *The Journal of Nervous and Mental Disease,* **186**: 769–775.

Goodman, J. (2013) *Paul Robeson: A watched man.* London: Verso.

Gordon, R. A. (1990) *Anorexia and bulimia: Anatomy of a social epidemic.* Oxford: Blackwell.

Gottesman, I. I., McGuffin, P. & Farmer, A. E. (1987) Clinical Genetics as Clue to the 'Real' Genetics of Schizophrenia (a Decade of Modest Gains While Playing for Time). *Schizophrenia Bulletin,* **13**: 23–47.

Hare, E. (1981). The Two Manias: A Study of the Evolution of the Modern Concept of Mania. *The British Journal of Psychiatry,* **138**: 89–99.

Harris, M., Chandran, S., Chakraborty, N. & Healy, D. (2005) The Impact of Mood Stabilizers on Bipolar Disorder: The 1890s and 1990s Compared. *History of Psychiatry,* **16(4)**: 423–434.

Harrison, P. J. (1999) The Neuropathology of Schizophrenia A Critical Review of the Data and Their Interpretation. *Brain,* **122**: 593–624.

Healy, D. (2010) From Mania to Bipolar Disorder. In: L. M. Yatham & M. Maj (eds) *Bipolar Disorder: Clinical and Neurobiological Foundations,* 1–7. Hoboken, NJ: Wiley-Blackwell.

Hershman, D. J. & Lieb, J. (1998) *Manic Depression and Creativity.* New York: Prometheus Books.

Hibberd, D. (2003) *Wilfred Owen: A New Biography.* London: Phoenix.

Hill, C. (1988) *God's Englishman: Oliver Cromwell and the English Revolution.* London: Peregrine Books.

Hillhouse, TM, Porter, JH (2015) A Brief History of the Development of Antidepressant drugs: From Monoamines to Glutamate, *Experimental and Clinical Psychopharmacology,* **23(1):** 1–21.

Hogsberg, C. (2010) CLR James and the Black Jacobins. *International Socialism Journal,* **126**: 95–120.

Hughes, J. C., (2011) Alzheimer's and Other Dementias. Oxford: Oxford University Press

HSCIC (Health & Social Care Information Centre) (2015) Mental Health Bulletin: Annual Statistics 2014–15, version 1.0.

HSE (Health and Safety Executive) (2018) Work–Related Stress, Depression or Anxiety Statistics in Great Britain 2018, retrieved from http://www.hse.gov.uk/statistics/causdis/stress.pdf.

Hughes, J. C., (2013) *Alzheimer's and Other Dementias.* Oxford: Oxford University Press.

Ihara, H. (2012) A Cold of the Soul: A Japanese Case of Disease Mongering in Psychiatry. *The International Journal of Risk and Safety in Medicine,* **24**: 115–120.

Jablensky, A. (2003). The Epidemiological Horizon. In: S. R. Hirsch & D. R. Weinberger (eds), 2nd Edition, *Schizophrenia*, 203–231. Oxford: Blackwell.

Jablensky, A., Sartorius, N., Ernberg, G., Anker, M., Korten, A., Cooper, J. E., Day, R. & Bertelson, A. (1992). Schizophrenia: Manifestations, Incidence and Course in Different Cultures. A WHO Ten-Country Study. *Psychological Medicine Supplement*, **20**: 1–7.

Jacobs Brumberg, J., (2000) *Fasting Girls: The History of Anorexia Nervosa*. New York: Vintage Books.

Johnson, S. L. (2003) Defining Bipolar Disorder. In: S. L. Johnson & R. L. Leahy (eds), *Psychological treatment of bipolar disorder*, 3–16. New York: Guilford Publications.

Jones, E., Hodgins Vermaas, R., Mccartney, H., Beech, C., Palmer, I., Hyams, K. & Wessely, S. (2003). Flashbacks and Post-Traumatic Stress Disorder: The Genesis of a 20th-Century Diagnosis. *British Journal of Psychiatry*, **182(2)**: 158–163.

Keller, R. (2001). Psychiatry in the British and French Empires, 1800–1962. *Journal of Social History*, **35**: 295–326.

Kennedy, N., Foy, F., Sherazi, R., McDonough, M. & McKeon, P. (2007). Long-term Social Functioning After Depression Treated by Psychiatrists: A Review. *Bipolar Disorders*, **9**: 25–37.

Kessler, R. C., Ruscio, A. M., Shear, K. & Wittchen, H. U. (2010) Epidemiology of Anxiety Disorders. *Current Topics in Behavioural Neurosciences*, **2**: 21–35.

Keynes, M. (2008) Balancing Newton's Mind: His Singular Behaviour and his Madness of 1692–1693. *Notes and Records of the Royal Society of London*, **62(3)**: 289–300.

Kleinman, A. & Cohen, A. (2001) A Global View of Depression from an Anthropological Perspective. In: A. Dawson & A. Tylee (eds), *Depression: Social and Economic Time Bomb*, 11–15, London: BMJ Books.

Kraepelin, E. (1896) Dementia Praecox. In: J. Cutting & M. Shepherd (eds), *The Clinical Roots of the Schizophrenia Syndrome*, 15–24, Cambridge: Cambridge University Press.

Kumari, V., Fannon, D., Peters, E. R., Ffytche, D. H., Sumich, A. L., Premkumar, P., Anilkumar, A. P., Andrew, C., Phillips, M. L., Williams, S. C. & Kuipers, E. (2011) Neural Changes Following Cognitive Behaviour Therapy for Psychosis: A Longitudinal Study. *Brain: A Journal of Neurology*, **134(Pt 8)**: 2396–2407.

Lam, D., Hayward, P., Watkins, E. R., Wright, K. & Sham, P. (2005) Relapse Prevention in Patients with Bipolar Disorder: Cognitive Therapy Outcome After two Years. *American Journal of Psychiatry*, **162**: 324–329.

Lam, D. H., Jones, S. H., Hayward, P. & Bright, J. A. (1999) *Cognitive Therapy for Bipolar Disorder. A Therapist's Guide to Concepts, Methods and Practice.* Chichester, England: John Wiley & Sons.

Lawrie, S. M. & Johnstone, E. C. (2004). Schizophrenia and related disorders. In: E. C. Johnstone, D. G. Cunningham Owens, S. M. Lawrie, M. Sharpe & C.P.L. Freeman (eds), *Companion to Psychiatric Studies,* 7th edition, 390–420, Edinburgh: Churchill Livingstone.

Leff, J. P. & Vaughn, C. (1980) The Interaction of Life-Events and Relatives' Expressed Emotion in Schizophrenia and Depressive Neurosis. *British Journal of Psychiatry,* **136**: 146–53.

Leudar, I. (2001) Voices in History. *Outlines,* **1**: 5–18.

Leudar, I. & Thomas, P. (2001) *Voices of Reason, Voices of Insanity.* London: Routledge.

Lewis, S. W. & Murray, R. M. (1987) Obstetric Complications, Neurodevelopmental Deviance, and Risk of Schizophrenia. *Journal of Psychiatric Research,* **21**: 413–421.

Liddle, P. F. & Barnes, T. R. (1990) Syndromes of Chronic Schizophrenia. *The British Journal of Psychiatry,* **157**: 558–561.

Linden, D. (2012) *The Biology of Psychological Disorders.* Basingstoke: Palgrave Macmillan.

Lloyd, T., Kennedy, N., Fearon, P., Kirkbride, Mallett, J. R., Leff, J., Holloway, J., Harrison, G., Dazzan, P., Morgan, K., Murray, R. M. & Jones, P. B. on behalf of the SOP study team (2005) Incidence of Bipolar Affective Disorder in Three UK Cities. *The British Journal of Psychiatry,* **186**: 126–131.

Lorch, M. (2006) Language and Memory Disorder in the Case of Jonathan Swift: Considerations on Retrospective Diagnosis. *Brain,* **129**: 3127–3137.

Mai, F. (2008) Emotion in Beethoven and His Music – Psychiatry in Music. *The British Journal of Psychiatry,* **193(3)**: 209.

Malhi, G. S., Tanious, M., Das, P., Coulston, C. M. & Berk, M. (2013) Potential Mechanisms of Action of Lithium in Bipolar Disorder. *CNS Drugs,* **27**: 135–153.

Malla, A. K., Cortese, L., Shaw, T. S. & Ginsberg, B. (1990). Life Events and Relapse in Schizophrenia. A One Year Prospective Study. *Social Psychiatry & Psychiatric Epidemiology,* **25**: 221–224.

Matsunaga, S., Kishi, T. & Iwata, N. (2015). Memantine Monotherapy for Alzheimer's Disease: A Systematic Review and Meta-Analysis. *PLOS One,* **10(4)**: 1–16.

Matthew, H.C.G. (1997) *Gladstone 1809–1898.* Oxford: Clarendon Press.

May, R. & Svanholmer, E. (2016) http://rufusmay.com/2016/02/09/getting-closer-to-the-personal-experience-of-psychosis/.

McColl, H. & McKenzie, K. & Bhui, (2008) Mental Healthcare of Asylum-Seekers and Refugees. *Advances in Psychiatric Treatment,* **14**: 452–459.

McDonald, C. & Murray, R. M. (2000). Early and Late Environmental Risk Factors for Schizophrenia. *Brain Research, Brain Research Review,* **31**: 130–137.

Mental Health Taskforce. (2016) The Five Year Forward View For Mental Health www.england.nhs.uk/wp-content/uploads/2016/02/Mental-Health-Taskforce-FYFV-final.pdf.

Miklowitz, D. J. & Johnson, S. L. (2006) The Psychopathology and treatment of Bipolar Disorder. *Annual Review of Clinical Psychology,* **2**: 199–235.

Mitchison, D. & Hay, P. J. (2014) The Epidemiology of Eating Disorders: Genetic, Environmental, and Societal Factors. *Clinical Epidemiology,* **6**: 89–97.

Morrison, A. P., Wells, A. & Nothard, S. (2000) Cognitive Factors in Predisposition to Auditory and Visual Hallucinations. *British Journal of Clinical Psychology,* **39**: 67–78.

Murphy, R., Straebler, S., Basden, S., Cooper, Z. & Fairburn, C. G. (2012) Interpersonal Psychotherapy for Eating Disorders. *Clinical Psychology and Psychotherapy,* **19**: 150–158.

Nardi, A. E. (2006) Some Notes on a Historical Perspective of Panic Disorder. *Jornal Brasileiro* de *Psiquiatria,* **55(2)**: 154–160.

NICE (2005) Obsessive-Compulsive Disorder and Body Dysmorphic Disorder: Treatment Clinical Guideline [CG31].

NICE (2017) Eating Disorders: Recognition and Treatment (NG 69).

NICE (2018) Post-Traumatic Stress Disorder (NG 116).

NHS Digital (2017) Prescriptions Dispensed in the Community, Statistics for England 2006–2016. Retrieved from http://digital.nhs.uk/catalogue/PUB30014.

Nuechterlein, K. H., Dawson, M. E. & Ventura, J. (1994) The Vulnerability-Stress Model of Schizophrenia Relapse: A Longitudinal Study. *Acta Psychiatrica Scandinavica Suppl,* **89**: 58–64.

Owen, M. J., Craddock, N. & O'Donovan, M. C. (2005) Schizophrenia: Genes at Last?. *TRENDS in Genetics,* **21**: 518–525.

Oyebode, F. (2010) 'A Crisis in my Mental History', from autobiography by John Stuart Mill. *Advances in Psychiatric Treatment,* **16**: 192.

Pearlman, J. (2013) A Year after Jovan Belcher's Final Act, Friends Offer Clues to Tragic Downfall. http://bleacherreport.com/articles/1861645-a-year-after-jovan-belchers-final-act-friends-offer-clues-to-tragic-downfall.

Peters, T. J. & Beveridge, A. (2010) The Madness of King George III: A Psychiatric Re-assessment. *History of Psychiatry,* **21**: 20–37.

Peters, T. J. & Willis, C. (2013) Mental Health Issues of Maria I of Portugal and Her Sisters: The Contributions of the Willis Family to the Development of Psychiatry. *History of Psychiatry,* **24**: 292–307.

Peterson, D. E. (1982) A Mad People's History of Madness. Pittsburgh, PA : University of Pittsburgh Press.

Phillips, P. & Labrow, J. (2004) Understanding Dual Diagnosis. Mind Publication. http://rcgnc.com/WellnesLibrary/Substance%20Use,%20 Dual%20Diagnosis%20&%20Addictions%20(Non-Substance)/ Understanding%20Dual%20Diagnosis%202007.pdf.

Pickover, C. A. (1999) *Strange Brains and Genius: The Secret Lives of Eccentric Scientists and Madmen.* New York: Quill, William Morrow.

Pietikainen, P. (2015) Madness a History. Abingdon: Routledge.

Porter, R. (1985) The Hunger of Imagination: Approaching Samuel Johnson's Melancholy. In: W.F. Bynum, R. Porter & M. Shepherd (eds), *The Anatomy of Madness,* vol **1**, 63–68. London: Routledge.

Porter, R. (1989) *A Social History of Madness.* London: Weidenfeld & Nicolson.

Porter, R. (2004) *Madmen: A Social History of Madhouses, Mad-Doctors & Lunatics.* Stroud, UK: Tempus Publishing.

Porter, R. (ed.) (2014) *George Cheyne: The English Malady* (1733), 1st edition. London: Routledge.

Post, F. (1994) Creativity and Psychopathology a Study of 291 World-Famous Men. *British Journal of Psychiatry,* **165**: 22–34.

Post, F. (1996) Verbal Creativity, Depression and Alcoholism an Investigation of One Hundred American and British Writers. *British Journal of Psychiatry,* **168**: 545–555.

Rachman., S. (1999) The Evolution of Cognitive Behaviour Therapy. In: D. M. Clark & C. G. Fairbairn (eds), *Science and Practice of Cognitive Behaviour Therapy,* 3–26. Oxford: Oxford University Press.

Rapoport, J. L., Addington, A. M., Frangou, S. & Psych, M.R.C. (2005) The Neurodevelopmental Model of Schizophrenia: Update 2005. *Molecular Psychiatry,* **10**: 434–449.

Ravindran, A. V. & da Silva, T. L. (2013) Complementary and Alternative Therapies as Add-on to Pharmacotherapy for Mood and Anxiety Disorders: A Systematic Review. *Journal of Affective Disorders,* **150**: 707–719.

Rayworth, B. B., Wise, L. A. & Harlow, B. L. (2004) Childhood Abuse and Risk of Eating Disorders in Women. *Epidemiology,* **15(3):** 271–278.

Read, J., Fosse, R., Moskowitz, A. & Perry, B. (2014) The Traumagenic Neurodevelopmental Model of Psychosis Revisited. *Neuropsychiatry,* **4**: 65–79.

Read, J., van Os, J., Morrison, A. P. & Ross, C. A. (2005) Childhood Trauma, Psychosis and Schizophrenia: A Literature Review with Theoretical and Clinical Implications. *Acta Psychiatrica Scandinavica*, **112**: 330–350.

Rector, N. A. & Seeman, M.V. (1992) Auditory Hallucinations in Women and Men. *Schizophrenia Research*, **7**: 233–236.

Redfield Jamison, K. (1996) *An Unquiet Mind: A Memoire of Moods and Madness*. London: Picador.

Roberts, J. S., (2000) *Siegfried Sassoon*. London: Richard Cohen Books.

Robinson, D. M. & Keating, G. M. (2006). 'Memantine: A Review of its Use in Alzheimer's Disease'. *Drugs*, **66(11)**: 1515–1534.

Romme, M.A.J., Honig, A., Noorthoorn., E. O. & Escher., D.M.A.C. (1992), Coping with Hearing Voices: An Emancipatory Approach. *British Journal of Psychiatry*, **161**: 99–103.

Rousseau, G. (2000) Depression's Forgotten Genealogy: Notes Towards a History of Depression. *History of Psychiatry*, **11**: 71–106.

RCP (Royal College of Psychiatrists) (2015) Information about ECT (Electro-Convulsive Therapy).

Ruggero, C. J., Zimmerman, M., Chelminski, I. & Young, D. (2010) Borderline Personality Disorder and the Misdiagnosis of Bipolar Disorder. *Journal of Psychiatric Research*, **44(6)**: 405–408.

Russell, G. (1979) Bulimia Nervosa: An Ominous Variant of Anorexia Nervosa. *Psychological Medicine*, **9**: 429–448.

Russell, G.F.M. (1997) The History of Bulimia Nervosa. In: D.M. Garner & P.E. Garfinkel (eds), *Handbook of Treatment for Eating Disorders*, 11–24, 2nd edition. New York: The Guilford Press.

Salkovskis, P. (2002) 'Review: Eye Movement Desensitization and Reprocessing is Not Better Than Exposure Therapies for Anxiety or Trauma'. *Evidence-Based Mental Health*, **5(1)**: 13.

Salkovskis, P. M. & Kirk, J. (1999) Obsessive Compulsive Disorder. In: D.M. Clark & C.G. Fairbairn (eds), *Science and Practice of Cognitive Behaviour Therapy*, 179–208. Oxford: Oxford University Press.

Salokangas, R.K.R. (2004) Gender and the Use of Neuroleptics in Schizophrenia. *Schizophrenia Research*, **66**: 41–49.

Schäfer, I. & Fisher, H. L. (2011) Childhood Trauma and Psychosis – What Is the Evidence? *Dialogues in Clinical Neuroscience*, **13(3)**: 360–365.

Schmidt, R.L. (2011) *Little Girl Blue: The Life of Karen Carpenter*. Chicago, IL: Chicago review Press.

Scull, A. (2015) *Madness in Civilisation*. London: Thanes & Hudson.

Sedgwick, P. (1987) *Psycho Politics*. London: Pluto Press.

Segman, R. H. & Lerer, B. (2000) Genetic and Causal Factors of Bipolar Disorder. In: J. C. Soares & S. Gershon (eds), *Bipolar Disorders Basic Mechanisms and Therapeutic Implications*, 31–48. New York: Marcel Dekker.

Shaji, K.S. (2009) Dementia Care in Developing Countries: The Road Ahead. *Indian Journal of Psychiatry*, **51**: s5–s7.

Shields, B. (2005) *Down Came the Rain: My Journey Through Postpartum Depression*. New York: Hyperion.

Shorter, E. (1997) *A History of Psychiatry: From the Era of the Asylum to the Age of Prozac*. New York: John Wiley & Sons.

Shorter, E. (2009) The History of Lithium Therapy. *Bipolar Disorder*, **11**: 4–9.

Showalter, E. (1997) *Hystories, Hysterical Epidemics and Modern Culture*. London: Picador.

Shtasel, D. L., Gur, R. E., Gallacher, F., Heimberg, C. & Gur, R. C. (1992) Gender Differences in the Clinical Expression of Schizophrenia. *Schizophrenia Research*, **7**: 225–231.

Slawenski, K. (2012) *J. D. Salinger: A Life*. New York: Random House.

Slobodin, O. & de Jong, J.T.V.M. (2015) Mental Health Interventions for Traumatised Asylum Seekers and Refugees: What Do We Know About Their Efficacy?. *International Journal of Social Psychiatry*, **61(1)**: 17–26.

Smink, F.R.E., van Hoeken, D. & Hoek, H. W. (2012) Epidemiology of Eating Disorders: Incidence, Prevalence and Mortality Rates. *Current Psychiatry Reports*, **14(4)**: 406–414.

Steinglass, J., Mayer, L. & Attia, E. (2016) Treatment of Restrictive Eating and Low-Weight Conditions, Including Anorexia Nervosa and Avoidant/Restrictive Food Intake Disorder. In: B.T. Walsh, E. Attia, D.R. Glasofer & R. Sysko (eds), *Handbook of Assessment and Treatment of Eating Disorders*, 259–278. Arlington, VA: American Psychiatric Association Publishing.

Stone, M. H. (1998) *Healing the Mind: A History of Psychiatry from Antiquity to the Present*. London: Pimlico.

Storr. A. (1993) *The Dynamics of Creation*. New York: Ballantine Books.

Strachan, A. (2018) *Dark Star: The Untold Story of Vivien Leigh*. London: Tauris.

Strakowski & Sax (2000) Secondary Mania a Model of the Pathophysiology of Bipolar Disorder? In: J. C. Soares & S. Gershon (eds), *Bipolar Disorders Basic Mechanisms and Therapeutic Implications*, 13–30. New York: Marcel Dekker.

Tekiner, H. (2015) Aretaeus of Cappadocia and his Treatises on Diseases. *Turkish Neurosurgery*, **25(3)**: 508–512.

Ter Heide, F., Mooren, T., Van de Schoot, R., De Jongh, A. & Kleber, R. (2016) Eye Movement Desensitisation and Reprocessing Therapy v. Stabilisation as Usual for Refugees: Randomised Controlled Trial. *British Journal of Psychiatry*, **209(4)**: 311–318.

Tivyside Advertiser (1870) www.welshlegalhistory.org/research-jacob-trial-report.php.

Toates, F. & Coschung-Toates, O. (2005) *Obsessive Compulsive Disorder: Practical, Tried and Tested Strategies to Overcome OCD*, London: Class Publishing.

Trimble, M. D. (1985) Post-Traumatic Stress Disorder: History of a Concept. In: C.R. Figley (ed.), *Trauma and Its Wake: The Study and Treatment of Post-Traumatic Stress Disorder*. New York: Brunner/Mazel. Revised from Encyclopedia of Psychology, R. Corsini, (ed.). New York: Wiley, 1984, 1994.

Turnbull, G. (2012) *Trauma. From Lockerbie to 7/7: How Trauma Affects Our Minds and How We Fight Back*. London: Corgi.

Vaughn, C. E., Sorensen Snyder, K., Jones, S., Freeman, W. B. & Falloon, I.R.H. (1984) Family Factors in Schizophrenic Relapse. Replication in California of British Research on Expressed Emotion. *Archives of General Psychiatry*, **41**: 1169–1177.

Veale, D. & Wilson, R. (2009) *Overcoming obsessive compulsive disorder*. London: Robinson.

Waddington, J. L., Buckley, P. F., Scully, P. J., Lane, A., O'Callaghan, E. & Larkin, C. (1998) Course of Psychopathology, Cognition and Neurobiological Abnormality in Schizophrenia: Developmental Origins and Amelioration by Antipsychotics? *Journal of Psychiatric Research,* **32**: 179–189.

Watt, N. F. (1972) Longitudinal Changes in the Social Behaviour of Children Hospitalized for Schizophrenia as Adults. *Journal of Nervous and Mental Disease,* **155**: 42–54.

Webb, T.E.F. (2006) 'Dottyville'—Craiglockhart War hospital and shell-shock treatment in the First World War. *Journal of the Royal Society of Medicine,* **99(7)**: 342–346.

Weinberger, D. A. (1987) Implications of Normal Brain Development for the Pathogenesis of Schizophrenia. *Archives of General Psychiatry,* **44**: 660–669.

Weinberger, D. R. & Marenco, S. (2003) Schizophrenia as a Neurodevelopmental Disorder. In: S. R. Hirsch & D. R. Weinberger (eds), *Schizophrenia*, 2nd edition, 326–348. Oxford: Blackwell.

Wells, A. & Butler, G. (1999) Generalized Anxiety Disorder. In: D.M. Clark, & C. G. Fairbairn (eds), *Science and Practice of Cognitive Behaviour Therapy*. Oxford: Oxford University Press.

Westbrook, D., Kennerley, H. & Kirk, J. (2008) *An Introduction to Cognitive Behaviour Therapy*. London: Sage.

White, K. S. & Barlow, D.H. (2004) Panic Disorder and Agoraphobia. In: D.H. Barlow (ed.), *Anxiety and Its Disorders*, 328–379. New York: The Guilford Press.

WHO, (1993) The ICD-10 Classification of Mental and Behavioural Disorders: Diagnostic Criteria for Research.

WHO (2001) Mental Disorders Fact Sheet N°396 updated October 2015. The World Health Report 2001 - Mental Health: New Understanding, New Hope.

WHO (2013) WHO Guidelines on Conditions Specifically Related to Stress www.who.int/mental_health/emergencies/stress_guidelines/en/.

WHO (2014) Preventing Suicide: A Global Imperative.

WHO (2017a) Fact Sheet No. 369 on Depression, updated February 2017. www.who.int/mediacentre/factsheets/fs369/en/.

WHO (2017b) Fact Sheet No. 362 on Dementia, updated December 2017. www.who.int/mediacentre/factsheets/fs362/en/.

WHO (2017c) mhGAP forum report. www.who.int/mental_health/mhgap/forum_report_2017/en/.

WHO (2018a) Fact Sheet on Mental Disorders. www.who.int/en/news-room/fact-sheets/detail/mental-disorders.

WHO (2018b) Suicide Key Facts. www.who.int/news-room/fact-sheets/detail/suicide.

WHO (2018c) The International Classification of Diseases, 11th Revision (ICD-11). https://icd.who.int/browse11/l-m/en.

Williams, J.M.G. (1999) Depression. In: D. M. Clark & C. G. Fairbairn (eds), *Science and Practice of Cognitive Behaviour Therapy*, 259–284. Oxford: Oxford University Press.

Wills, G. L. (2003) Forty Lives in the Bebop Business: Mental Health in a Group of Eminent Jazz Musicians. *British Journal of Psychiatry, 183*: 255–259.

Wilson, A. (2000) On the History of Disease-Concepts: The Case of Pleurisy. *History of Science, 38*: 271–319.

Wing, J. K. (1978) *Reasoning About Madness*. Oxford: Oxford University Press.

Wing, J. K. & Agrawal, N. (2003) Concepts and Classification of Schizophrenia. In: S.R. Hirsch & D.R. Weinberger (eds), *Schizophrenia*, 2nd edition, 3–14. Oxford: Blackwell.

Index

Acetylcholinesterase inhibitors
   (AChEI)
treatment for dementia, 69
Alcohol
   Alastair Campbell and, 61
   alcoholism and writers, 130
   Carrie Fisher and, 138
   dual diagnosis *see* pages, 142–149
   Elton John and, 92
   George Trosse and, 106
   Hemmingway and, 57
   Makes panic disorder worse, 30
   risk factor for relapse in Bipolar
      disorder, 141
   Rita Hayworth and, 67
Alzheimer, Alois, 62
Alzheimer's disease *see* Chapter 3
   Dementia, 62–68
   Treatments for, 68
Anderson, Hans Christian and OCD,
   24–25
Antidepressants
   For anorexia, 88–89
   Bipolar Disorder, 140
   For Bulimia, 92
   For Depression, 47–48
   For OCD, 28
   For Panic Disorder, 32
   Not recommended for PTSD, 44
   Serendipitous discover of, 59
   For Social Phobia, 19
Antipsychiatry
   campaigns for better treatment,
      120–121
   critique of ECT, 57–58

Antipsychotics
   To treat anorexia or psychosis,
      118–120
   To treat Bipolar Disorder, 127
   side effects, 119
Antiquity
   madness in, 10, 12, 14, 48, 66, 90
Anorexia *see* Chapter 4
   Eating Disorders, 74–77
   Fasting Girls, 80–83
   Modern conception, of 84
   Religious fasting, 77–80
   Treatment, 88–89
Anxiety *see* Chapter 1
   associated with dual diagnosis,
      146
   generalised anxiety ,7
   Health and Safety Executive
      figures for work-related stress,
      depression and anxiety 2018,
      54
   Jane Fonda and, 91
   Panic Disorder, 8–9, 29–32
   As a psychological symptom of
      anorexia, 88
   As a psychological symptom of
      dementia, 64a
   social anxiety disorder, 15–21
   As a side effect of Mertrazol, 56
   As a symptom of depression, 47
Aretaeus of Cappadocia
   early description of Bipolar
      disorder 125,
Asylums
   the era of, 108–115

Barton, Clara
American Nurse, founder of the American Red Cross and social anxiety disorder, 18
Beers, Clifford, 114–115
Beethoven, Ludwig van
And Bipolar Disorder, 134–135
Mental health and alcohol abuse, 143
Bethlehem Hospital, also Bedlam
and government commission, 110
First psychiatric hospital, 109
Bipolar Disorder *see* Chapter 6, 123
Causes of, 128–129
Creativity and bipolar disorder, 129–131
Development of the concept of bipolar disorder, 125–128
Treatments for Bipolar, 139–141
Bleuler, Eugene
and Schizophrenia, 96–97
meets Nijinsky, 116
Bruch, Hilde, and Anorexia, 84–85, 89
Bulimia nervosa, 89–92
Treatments for Bulimia, 92–93
Burton, Robert
Anatomy of Melancholia, 22, 48, 105
And melancholy, 12–13

Cade, John
rediscovery of Lithium, 139
Campbell, Alastair
challenging stigma, 61
problems with alcohol and depression, 141
Carpenter, Karen
and anorexia, 85–86
Catherine of Siena, 78–79
Chronic Traumatic Encephalopathy (CTE), 65
Christie, Agatha
and Depression, 54–55

Churchill, Winston
and alcohol, 146
and dementia, 66
and depression, 52
Cognitive Behaviour Therapy (CBT)
for Anorexia, 89
for Bipolar Disorder, 140
for Bulimia, 92–93
for Depression, 58, 59
for Panic Disorder, 31–32
for Psychosis, 101
for PTSD, 43–45
For Social anxiety disorder, 19–20
Cromwell, Oliver
and Depression, 50–51

Dementia *see* Chapter 3, 62–70
Causes of, 63–65
Demographics of, 63–64
Medications used to treat Dementia, 69
Sports people and, 64–65
Treatments for Dementia, 68–70
Dementia Praecox *see* Schizophrenia, 96
Depression *see* Chapter 2, 46–61
causes of, 47–48
cricketers and, 53–54
Demographics, 1, 46
development of the concept, 48–50
and Melancholy, 11
politicians and, 52–53
Treatments for, 58–60
and stigma, 46–47, 61
Women and, 60
writers and, 54
Dickens, Charles, 134–135

Eating Disorders; *see also* Chapter 4; Anorexia; Bulimia
Demographics, 72
genetic influences, 74

Electroconvulsive Therapy, (ECT)
  Carrie Fisher is treated with it, 138
  critique of, 57–58
  Ernest Hemmingway is treated
    with it, 57
  history of, 56–57
  Paul Robeson is treated with it, 56
  Vivien Leigh is treated with it,
    136–137
  women more likely to receive it, 60
Exorcism
  as response to demonic possession
    in China, 11
  Christoph Haizmann has an
    exorcism, 106
  Christian response to perceived
    demonic possession, 12, 14, 106
Eye Movement Desensitisation and
    Reprocessing (EMDR) for PTSD,
    43
  critique of, 43–44
Eden, Anthony
  Anxiety, drug and alcohol misuse
    whilst Prime Minister, 147

Fasting Girls, 80–83
Freud, Sigmund
  and Anxiety, 30
  influence on practices at
    Craiglockhart, 38
  views on anorexia, 83–84
  views on creativity, 130
  views on psychosis, 115
Fry, Stephen, 137–138
Fisher, Carrie
  and Bipolar disorder, 138

Galen (Aelius Galenus)
  and decline in mental faculties, 65
  decline of Galenic medicine with
    the enlightenment, 108
  survival of the Galenic tradition
    in Islamic medicine, 103

  writings on Mania and
    Melancholy, 11–13
George III
  and Bipolar Disorder, 131–132
Gladstone, William Ewart
  and Hypomania, 135–136
Gull, William
  and the description of Anorexia,
    74–77

Haizmann, Christoph
  visions and pact with the devil,
    106–107
Hemmingway, Ernest
  Dual Diagnosis, 145
  ECT and suicide, 57
Hitler, Adolph
  hysterical reaction to combat, 15
Hippocrates
  first written reference to phobias, 9
Hughes, Howard and OCD, 25–26
Hysteria
  conceptualisation of, 14–15
  as an explanation for anorexia,
    83

Imipramine, discovery of
    antidepressants, 59
Insulin Coma Therapy for psychosis,
    115–116
Interpersonal therapy (IPT) for
    depression, 58
  for anorexia, 89
  for Bipolar disorder, 140
  for bulimia, 93

Jacobs, Sarah fasting
    girl, 81–82
Jamison, Kay Redfield personal
    experience of Bipolar disorder,
    137
Johnson, Samuel
  and OCD, 23–25

Kempe Marjorie, 104–105
Kraepelin, Emile
  and Alzheimer's disease,
    62–63
  classification of mental disorders,
    126–127
  and dementia praecox/
    schizophrenia, 96–97

Leigh, Vivien, 136–137
Lithium treatment for Bipolar
  disorder, 139–140
Lloyd George, David
  and depression, 52–53
Lobotomy, 117
Luther, Martin
  and OCD, 22–23

MacDonald, Ramsay
  and dementia, 67
Mania and humoural theory, 11
  in Bipolar disorder, 124–128,
    131–133,
  link to melancholy, 48
  treatments for, 139
Melancholia and depression, 48,
    50–51
  linked to mania, 125–126
Mood stabilisers, 140
May, Rufus, 121

Nijinsky, Vaslav, 116
Newton, Isaac, 133

Obsessive Compulsive Disorder
  (OCD), 21–29
Owen, Wilfred
  and 'Shell shock', 36–39

Perceval, John
  advocate for mental health
    reform, 110–112
Phobias, 16–17

Pinel, Philippe
  and Dementia, 66
  mental health reforms, 110
Pitt, William (the elder)
  and Depression, 133–134
Poe, Edgar Allen, 144
Psychosis *see* Chapter 5
  convulsive therapy for, 56
  Glass delusion, 105
  and Schizophrenia, 95
  social and environmental
    influences, 100
  Trauma, 101–102
  treatments for, 115–122
PTSD *see* Chapter 1
  Anxiety Disorders, 33–45

Ridley, Arnold
  and PTSD, 39–40
Robeson, Paul, 55–56
Romme, Marius
  Hearing Voices Network, 121
Rossetti, Dante Gabriel
  mental health, drugs and alcohol,
    144–145

Salinger, JD and PTSD, 40
Sassoon, Siegfried at Craiglockhart
  and PTSD, 36–39
Schizophrenia *see* Chapter 5
  aetiology of psychosis, 99–102
  criticisms of the diagnostic
    category, 95–96
  development of the concept, 96–97
  gender differences, 98
  historical conceptions, 102–104
  Psychosis, difficulty of
    retrospective diagnosis, 4
  trauma and psychosis, 101
  treatments, 115–122
Sexton, Anne, 145–146
  dual diagnosis and suicide
Shell Shock, 36–38

Simpson, Joe and Touching the
    Void, 41
Socrates and his Daemon, 102–102
Stigma, 46
    as a barrier to effective care, 48
    challenging the stigma of
        depression, 61
    contemporary challenges to it,
        137–138
Storr Anthony, The Dynamics of
    Creation, 130–131
Suicide
    and Bipolar Disorder, 123
    Depression, 47
    high rates in cricketers, 53–54
    high rates in writers, 54
    prevalence rate of, 1

Swift, Jonathan, 66

Tesla, Nikola and OCD, 26
Trauma; *see also* PTSD; CTE
    Psychosis, 101

Williams, Tennessee, 145
Willis Thomas and Hysteria, 14
Women
    Anorexia, 84–85
    and anxiety disorders, 6
    and Depression, 46, 60
    and Eating Disorders, 72–80
    and Panic Disorder, 29,
    and Schizophrenia, 98
Wright Orville, 18–19